RECENT ADVANCES IN HEMATOLOGY RESEARCH

VENOUS THROMBOSIS

RISK FACTORS, MANAGEMENT AND COMPLICATIONS

RECENT ADVANCES IN HEMATOLOGY RESEARCH

Additional books in this series can be found on Nova's website under the Series tab.

Additional e-books in this series can be found on Nova's website under the e-book tab.

RECENT ADVANCES IN HEMATOLOGY RESEARCH

VENOUS THROMBOSIS

RISK FACTORS, MANAGEMENT AND COMPLICATIONS

CAROLINE H. GUTMANN
EDITOR

NOVA BIOMEDICAL

New York

For permission to use material from this book please contact us:
Telephone 631-231-7269; Fax 631-231-8175
Web Site: http://www.novapublishers.com

Library of Congress Cataloging-in-Publication Data

ISBN: 978-1-63117-293-9

Library of Congress Control Number: 2014931439

Published by Nova Science Publishers, Inc. † New York

Contents

Preface

Thrombophilias can be defined as a group of inherited or acquired disorders that increase the risk of developing thrombosis. Venous thromboembolism (VT) is considered a multifactorial disease produced by a sum of risk factors that predispose to the thrombotic event. This predisposition includes genetic and acquired defects. Thrombosis can occur in any section of the venous system, but commonly manifests as deep vein thrombosis of the leg and pulmonary embolism. Major complications of venous thrombosis are a disabling post-thrombotic syndrome, pulmonary hypertension, and sudden death duo to a pulmonary embolism and therefore, it poses a burden on health economy. Venous thrombosis is a common clinical challenge for doctors of all disciplines, as it is a complex multicausal disease. This books discusses in further detail the many complications and risk factors caused by venous thrombosis.

Chapter 1 - Breast cancer is the most common malignancy in females, after skin cancer, with lifetime incidence of 12.4% and the second most common cause of cancer related deaths among women. Venous thromboembolic (VTE) events have been found to affect 0.16 to 2.3% of breast cancer patients and are associated with increased mortality. Nearly all breast cancer patients require mastectomy or lumpectomy as part of the treatment regimen and many of these patients also undergo reconstruction, either immediate or delayed. Risk factors associated with VTE include advanced cancer stage, prolonged operative time, inpatient hospitalization, immediate reconstruction, chronic medical comorbidities, venous catheterization, age, obesity, and tamoxifen or chemotherapy use. This chapter will focus on VTE complications that arise from surgical treatment, mastectomy, and breast reconstruction, in breast cancer patients. Identifying risk factors will help guide physicians to improved prevention practices and hopefully a standardized VTE prophylaxis protocol for breast cancer patients.

Chapter 2 - The clinical significance of isolated calf vein thrombosis (ICVT) is controversial. It has not been adequately studied and its diagnostic and management guidelines are not universally similar. The majority of ICVTs are asymptomatic, diagnosed on screening ultrasound duplex sonography and do not propagate above the knee. A smaller portion of ICVTs are symptomatic and may propagate this subgroup can cause significant morbidity and even mortality. Management of ICVT differs among physicians and institutions. Some therapeutically anticoagulate, whereas some advise chemical and/or mechanical prophylaxis. Some physicians advise close surveillance with repetitive duplex scanning. For patients that are at high risk for clot propagation short term theoretic anticoagulation is recommended.

Chapter 3 – The incidence of deep venous thrombosis (DVT) in the surgical population varies by type of patient and surgical procedure, contributing an unknown percentile of the overall estimated 250,000 DVTs annually.

Most DVTs are proximal and are found above the knee in the iliac, femoral, or popliteal veins. Those found below the knee, in any of the three groups of paired deep calf veins, are typically considered of less clinical significance. Upper extremity DVTs, in the axillary and subclavian veins, account for 5% of DVTs and are seen most often in the surgical patient associated with indwelling catheters or in patients with malignancy; 30% of these DVTs are estimated to lead to pulmonary embolism (PE). Risk factors for DVT include advanced age, malignancy, immobilization, trauma, oral contraceptives, hormone replacement, pregnancy, obesity, neurologic or cardiac disease, prolonged travel, and inflammatory states. A recent review of 1,485 spinal surgery patients found similar factors such as active malignancy, prior DVT or PE, estrogen replacement therapy, and renal disease to be significant on univariate analysis.

Interestingly, on multivariate analysis, estrogen replacement therapy and discharge to a rehabilitation facility had the strongest correlations as risk factors for DVT or PE.

A high index of suspicion is necessary for early diagnosis of this condition. Signs and symptoms include pain, edema usually of the calf or ankle, and warmth or erythema of the skin over the thrombosis. More than 50% of DVTs are asymptomatic and found solely on imaging. Duplex ultrasound imaging is highly sensitive and specific. Laboratory tests such as

D-dimer can be useful adjuncts in making the diagnosis of DVT, although this is not as sensitive or specific for the disease as duplex ultrasonography.

The goal of DVT treatment is to reduce the risk of PE, decrease extension of DVT, and prevent the almost 30% recurrence rate of an untreated DVT. Systemic anticoagulation is the mainstay of treatment in patients diagnosed with DVT and PE. Catheter directed pharmacologic thrombolysis is another option that is thought to preserve valve function. Inferior vena cava (IVC) filter placement is another aspect of DVT treatment.

Chapter 4 – Superficial thrombophlebitis is defined as inflammation and thrombosis of a vein near the skin's surface. Most studies underestimate the occurrence of superficial thormbophlebitis and although the greater or lesser saphenous veins are the most commonly affected veins, this disease can occur at any part of the body.

This condition is often associated with a long term intravenous (IV) catheter and is differentiated from septic thrombophlebitis by the absence of systemic signs of infection. Risk factors include recent venous catheterization, a history of previous superficial venous thrombosis, DVT or PE, recent surgery, trauma, pregnancy, high dose estrogen therapy, immobilization, malignancy, varicose veins, obesity, or intravenous drug abuse.

Superficial thrombophlebitis remains a clinical diagnosis. Symptoms include localized pain and warmth over the site and patients will present with tenderness to palpation, induration, and erythema over a palpable cord. It is noted that superficial thrombophlebitis coexists with DVT in up to 53% of cases and PE in up to 33% of cases. Superficial thrombo-phlebitis can progress rapidly to venous thromboembolism (VTE) in as much as 15% of cases.

Even though most times superficial thrombophlebitis will resolve on its own, it is not considered to be self limited and complications can occur. These include extension from a superficial vein to a deep vein, postphlebitic syndrome, chronic DVTs, suppurative thrombophlebilitis and septic thrombophlebitis.

The aim of treatment is to alleviate symptoms and prevent extension to deep veins. The mainstay of treatment consists of extremity elevation, warm compresses, and the use of non-steroidal anti-inflammatory drugs (NSAID). Most patients respond to this conservative management regime with symptom resolution or improvement in 7-10 days. There is some evidence that shows the use of subtherapeutic doses of low molecular weight heparin can help in prevention of extension of superficial thrombophlebitis to DVT but there are no large multicenter trials to support this and make it standard of care.

Chapter 5 – Thrombophilias can be defined as a group of inherited or acquired disorders that increase the risk of developing thrombosis. Venous thromboembolism (VT) is considered a multifactorial disease produced by a sum of risk factors that predispose to the thrombotic event. This predisposition includes genetic and acquired defects. VT is one of the major public health problems worldwide, contributing to an estimated >500,000 deaths in Europe each year, with a mortality rate of 10%. The risk of recurrence is about 6% per year, and post-thrombotic disease occurs within the next 5 years following a VT event in about 25% of patients. VT is a common multifactorial disease, with both established environmental and genetic risk factors.

The genetic basis of the VT is only partially known, and thrombophilia can only explain around 50% of the thrombotic events. Hence, the known risk factors, together with yet unknown alterations in any component of the haemostatic system, may allow us to further clarify the underlying mechanism of VT. The known genetic risk factors confer a poor relative VT risk, altogether can only explain about 5% of the VT heritability.

The identification of disease-associated VT genes suspected to be involved in the physiopathology of the disease could help to define its genetic determinants.

Moreover, the recent availability of high-throughput genotyping technologies and their application in the framework of genome-wide association studies (GWAS) have enabled the identification of novel susceptibility loci. From 1965 to 2013, 16 genes/loci have been robustly associated with the susceptibility to VT, most of them affecting the coagulation cascade. In addition to the well-known established susceptibility genes for VT: *F5*, *F2*, *FGG*, *PROC*, *PROS*, *SERPINC1*, and ABO blood group, new emerging susceptibility loci have arisen: *C4BPA/C4BPB*, *F11*, *G6P*, *HIVEP1*, *KNG1*, *STXBP5*, *TCN2*, *VWF*. However, independent case-control studies are needed to confirm the association with the disease for these emerging genes. This chapter summarizes the current information on the role of genetic risk factors for venous thrombosis.

Chapter 6 – The annual incidence of venous thrombosis varies from 40 per 100,000 to 250 per 100,000 in different populations. Thrombosis can occur in any section of the venous system, but commonly manifests as deep vein thrombosis of the leg and pulmonary embolism. Major complications of venous thrombosis are a disabling post-thrombotic syndrome, pulmonary hypertension, and sudden death duo to a pulmonary embolism and therefore, it poses a burden on health economy. Venous thrombosis is a common clinical challenge for doctors of all disciplines, as it is a complex multicausal disease.

Hereditary conditions account for ~60% of all the thrombosis incidents and a number of genetic risk factors have been identified so far. Acquired risk factors may contribute to variations within and between individuals. Diagnosis of thrombosis is not difficult with the development of imaging techniques. However, the most important steps for diagnosis are etiology analyzes and genetic tests, which are useful for assessments of duration of anticoagulant therapy and prevention for thrombosis.

Chapter 7 – Thrombotic diseases develop as the result of multiple interactions between non-genetic and genetic risk factors. The known atherogenic risk factors played an important role as predictors in the development of the thrombotic diseases in the present female case-control study. The most important non-genetic risk factors found among the female patients are: age, hypercholesterolemia, DM, use of oral contraception, obesity, and fibrinogen levels. Moreover, the stratified effect of some of these factors according to the age of the patients is relevant for clinical risk assessment. Associations between the risk of venous thrombosis (VT) and genetic polymorphisms have been established. Some of these polymorphisms are highly prevalent in Caucasians, but there is a significant geographic variation in their prevalence among different populations. The MTHFR C677T (rs1801133), are analyses in females with stroke, venous thrombosis and myocardial infarction in a case-control study. The C677TMTHFR mutation were detected in 149 patients and 113 controls (P=0,001). In the present study, the results showed that hypercholesterolemia, diabetes mellitus, and elevated levels of fibrinogen were present in the younger group as risks factors. Family history of thrombotic event (TE) was statistically significantly associated among the older female group. Median values of total fibrinogen were significantly higher in the cases compared with the control group. The small numbers of carriers of these risk factors require a note of caution on any conclusion. The present data suggest that MTHFR C677T genotype may be an important factor in the life of female patients at risk of developing TE or cardiovascular disease , p=0,001 between cases and controls groups . Folic acid supplementation of foods is necessary (and mandatory in Costa Rica) before and during women's reproductive phase. However, our data presented suggest that a case for efforts to ensure a good intake of this vitamin in the postmenopausal phase. Especially if the high prevalence of the MTHFR 677T homozygosity and of classic risk factors in the Costa Rican population are taken into account. Further studies with more patients are necessary for final conclusions for these interactions to be drawn.

Chapter 8 - Cerebral Venous thrombosis (CVT) accounts for nearly 1-2% of all strokes. Isolated cortical vein thrombosis (ICVT), a subtype of CVT, without sinus or great venous involvement is rare. It is often difficult to diagnose due to its varied clinical and imaging features. Hence, the available literature largely comprises of single center case series. The common presenting symptoms of ICVT are focal seizures, vaguely defined focal neurological deficits and visual disturbances. Headache and raised intracranial pressure are relatively uncommon. The underlying conditions which may predispose to ICVT are the same as described for typical CVT. However, rare associations of ICVT include lumbar puncture, Hodgkin's disease, nephrotic syndrome, vasculitis, inflammatory bowel disease and amyloid angiopathy. With a high index of suspicion, neuroimaging is essential for direct visualization of the thrombus, localized hemorrhage or small venous infarction. Visualization of thrombosed cortical vein (the cord sign) is observed infrequently. Management guidelines are not well established. However, initial anticoagulation with heparin followed by oral anticoagulation for 6-12 months remains the recommended guideline for treatment of ICVT. The prognosis is generally good with radiological resolution in most cases. In this review, we present the clinical spectra, etiopathogenesis, neuroimaging features and management options in ICVT patients.

In: Venous Thrombosis
Editor: Caroline H. Gutmann

ISBN: 978-1-63117-293-9

Chapter 1

Venous Thromboembolism in Oncologic and Reconstructive Breast Surgery

Solmaz Niknam Leilabadi, M.D., M.H.A., Hyuma A. Leland, M.D., Vinaya Soundararajan, B.S. and Alex K. Wong, M.D., F.A.C.S.[*]

Division of Plastic and Reconstructive Surgery, Department of Surgery, Keck School of Medicine of USC, Los Angeles, CA, US

Abstract

Breast cancer is the most common malignancy in females, after skin cancer, with lifetime incidence of 12.4% and the second most common cause of cancer related deaths among women. Venous thromboembolic (VTE) events have been found to affect 0.16 to 2.3% of breast cancer patients and are associated with increased mortality. Nearly all breast cancer patients require mastectomy or lumpectomy as part of the treatment regimen and many of these patients also undergo reconstruction, either immediate or delayed. Risk factors associated with VTE include advanced cancer stage, prolonged operative time, inpatient hospitalization, immediate reconstruction, chronic medical comorbidities, venous catheterization, age, obesity, and tamoxifen or chemotherapy use.

[*] corresponding author, email: alex.wong@med.usc.edu.

This chapter will focus on VTE complications that arise from surgical treatment, mastectomy, and breast reconstruction, in breast cancer patients. Identifying risk factors will help guide physicians to improved prevention practices and hopefully a standardized VTE prophylaxis protocol for breast cancer patients.

Introduction

Venous thromboembolism (VTE) occurs rarely, but when unrecognized it can lead to significant morbidity and mortality. VTE encompasses both pulmonary embolism (PE) and deep vein thrombosis (DVT). Acute mortality from VTE is the result of embolic migration of a DVT into the pulmonary artery. In the general population, age-adjusted incidence of VTE is approximately 1 in 1000 people. [1] In cancer patients, this risk can be increased up to seven-fold, depending on the type of cancer. [1] VTE is preventable if high risk individuals are given prophylactic anti-coagulation.

Breast cancer is the most common form of cancer, aside from skin cancer, in women, occurring in 1 out of 8 women in the United States. [2] A review of the literature indicates that the risk of VTE in breast cancer ranges from 0.16 to 2.3%. Interestingly, while the incidence of VTE in breast cancer is lower than other forms of cancer, those who actually develop VTE in this setting have a very high mortality rate. [1,3] In fact, circulatory system disease, including VTE, is the second most common cause of death in breast cancer patients, following cancer itself. [4] Patients may also develop chronic symptoms from VTE, such as severe pain, edema, ulceration, post-phlebitic syndrome, and chronic thromboembolic pulmonary hypertension, leading to significant morbidity and decreased quality of life.

Until recently, the low incidence of VTE in breast cancer precluded researchers from understanding more about the disease. However, the development of regional and national registries and databases has given new insight into the disease process and risk factors for VTE in breast cancer patients. Because VTE is a preventable complication that has significant, life-threatening consequences, it is important to determine the risk factors and establish a standardized protocol for prophylaxis. Breast cancer treatments, including chemotherapy, hormonal therapy, radiotherapy, the placement of central venous catheters, and surgery itself greatly increase the likelihood of developing VTE. [5] To reduce this risk, some physicians have integrated routine use of pharmacologic anticoagulant prophylaxis, graded antithrombotic elastic compression stockings, and intermittent pneumatic compression devices into their practice. [5] Early ambulation and mechanical prophylaxis have shown to be best methods of VTE prevention for the majority of low risk breast cancer patients. [6]

This chapter will focus on VTE complications that arise from mastectomy and breast reconstruction in breast cancer patients. Identifying risk factors will help guide physicians to improved prevention practices and hopefully a standardized VTE prophylaxis protocol for breast cancer patients.

Venous Thromboembolism in Mastectomy Patients

The incidence of VTE in breast cancer patients ranges from 0.16-2.3%, [3,5] which is low compared to other malignancies; however, the high incidence of breast cancer translates to nearly 5,300 cases of VTE per year in U.S. breast cancer patients alone. VTE is a poor prognostic factor, correlating with worse overall survival and disease specific survival, in age, cancer type, stage, and surgical procedure matched patients. [7] In one series of 89 patients who underwent a modified radical mastectomy, two out of the five patients who developed a DVT also developed a PE, one of which died. [8] This increased mortality finding was also supported in a review of over 108,000 breast cancer patients that demonstrated a 2.3-fold increased risk of death over two years in breast cancer patients with VTE. [9] The American College of Chest Physicians (ACCP) publishes comprehensive evidence based clinical practice guidelines for antithrombotic therapy and prevention of thrombosis in medical and surgical patients. [10] The guidelines for general and abdominal surgery patients are summarized in Table 1; however, there are no evidence-based guidelines specifically for plastic and reconstructive surgery patients as there is a lack of randomized trials investigating VTE in these patients.[10] Clinically, despite well reported increased risk and associated mortality in breast cancer patients with VTE, a survey of over 600 reconstructive breast surgeons revealed only 25% of surgeons reported compliance with the ACCP guidelines on thromboprophylaxis. [11] Failure to meet the standard of care in VTE prevention has reinforced the need for all surgeons to assess whether VTE prophylaxis is indicated on a per patient basis. The Caprini risk assessment model (RAM), along with recent studies that improve our recognition of risk factors that confer greater risk of VTE in breast cancer patients, can help guide the decision to initiate VTE prophylaxis.

Table 1. Summary of ACCP recommendations for patients undergoing general or abdominal-pelvic surgeries. Recommendations compiled from American College of Chest Physicians recommendations. [10]

Level of risk for VTE	Recommendation
Very low risk (Caprini Score 0)	No specific pharmacologic or mechanical prophylaxis other than early ambulation
Low risk (Caprini score 1-2)	Mechanical prophylaxis, preferably IPC, over no prophylaxis
Moderate risk (Caprini score 3-4) who are NOT at high risk for major bleeding complication	LMWH, low dose UH, or mechanical prophylaxis, preferably IPC, over no prophylaxis
Moderate risk (Caprini score 3-4) who are at high risk for major bleeding complication or those in whom the consequences of bleeding are thought to be particularly severe	Mechanical prophylaxis, preferably IPC, over no prophylaxis
High risk (Caprini score ≥5) who are NOT at high risk for major bleeding complication	LMWH or low dose UH over no prophylaxis, suggest mechanical prophylaxis with elastic stockings or IPC should be added to pharmacologic prophylaxis
High risk undergoing abdominal or pelvic surgery for cancer who are not otherwise at high risk for major bleeding complications	Extended-duration pharmacologic prophylaxis (4 weeks) with LMWH over limited-duration prophylaxis
High risk undergoing abdominal or pelvic surgery who are at high risk for major bleeding complication or those in whom the consequences of bleeding are thought to be particularly severe	Mechanical prophylaxis, preferably IPC, over no prophylaxis until risk of bleeding diminishes and pharmacologic prophylaxis may be initiated
High risk in whom both LMWH and UH are contraindicated or unavailable and who are not at high risk for major bleeding complications	Low-dose aspirin, fondaparinux, or mechanical prophylaxis, preferably IPC, over no prophylaxis

LMWH = low molecular weight heparin, UH = unfractionated heparin, IPC = intermittent pneumatic compression

Caprini Risk Assessment Model

The Caprini RAM was developed in an effort to risk stratify medical and surgical patients based on risk factors derived from clinical experience and published data. Several iterations of the Caprini RAM have emerged since it was first reported in 1991, [12] and recently, the 2005 Caprini RAM (Figure 1) was found to most accurately risk stratify plastic and reconstructive surgery patients. [12] The Caprini RAM has been validated in a variety of patient populations, including plastic and reconstructive surgery, [13] general surgery, urology, otolaryngology, [14] vascular surgery, and medical inpatients [15].

The Caprini score is calculated by assessing a point value to VTE risk factors in general categories of age, obesity, surgical operation, medical comorbidities, mobility, and hereditary risk. Point values are then stratified by range into very low, low, moderate, high, and super-high risk. Until 2012, ACCP guidelines did not make recommendations on plastic and reconstructive surgery patients and currently do not specifically address breast surgery. Therefore, consensus guidelines presented herein are based on the 2011 American Society of Plastic Surgery (ASPS) VTE Task Force, which specifically addresses VTE prophylaxis recommendations for plastic and reconstructive surgery patients.

The ASPS VTE Task Force recommends all inpatients undergoing surgery under general anesthesia be assessed by the Caprini RAM or an equivalent RAM. Physicians should also consider whether outpatients undergoing general anesthesia should also be assessed. While ASPS does not specifically give recommendations on very low and low risk patients, ACCP [16] and leaders in VTE risk assessment modeling, including Caprini [17] and Pannucci, [13] have recommended early ambulation for patients with a Caprini score of zero, and intermittent pneumatic compression (IPC) for patients with a Caprini score of 1-2. Low risk patients have approximately a 1.5% risk of VTE over 60 days without any chemical prophylaxis. In moderate and high risk patients with a Caprini score of 3-6, ASPS recommends low molecular weight heparin (LMWH) or unfractionated heparin (UH) if not contraindicated by bleeding risk. Additionally, patients should receive concomitant IPC, as it has been shown to synergistically enhance VTE chemical prophylaxis. [18,19] Pannucci, et al., [20] have reported that super-high risk patients with a Caprini score over 8 have a VTE risk of 11.3% over 60 days, without perioperative administration of pharmacologic VTE prophylaxis. Therefore, ASPS VTE Task Force guidelines recommend LMWH or UH administration for 4 weeks after surgery when the Caprini score is greater than 7.

Choose All That Apply

Each Risk Factor Represents 1 Point

- Age 41-60 years
- Minor surgery planned
- History of prior major surgery (< 1 month)
- Varicose veins
- History of inflammatory bowel disease
- Swollen legs (current)
- Obesity (BMI > 25)
- Acute myocardial infarction
- Congestive heart failure (< 1 month)
- Sepsis (< 1 month)
- Serious lung disease incl. pneumonia (< 1 month)
- Abnormal pulmonary function (COPD)
- Medical patient currently at bed rest
- Other risk factors________________

Each Risk Factor Represents 2 Points

- Age 60-74 years
- Arthroscopic surgery
- Malignancy (present or previous)
- Major surgery (> 45 minutes)
- Laparoscopic surgery (> 45 minutes)
- Patient confined to bed (> 72 hours)
- Immobilizing plaster cast (< 1 month)
- Central venous access

Each Risk Factor Represents 5 Points

- Elective major lower extremity arthroplasty
- Hip, pelvis or leg fracture (< 1 month)
- Stroke (< 1 month)
- Multiple trauma (< 1 month)
- Acute spinal cord injury (paralysis)(< 1 month)

Each Risk Factor Represents 3 Points

- Age over 75 years
- History of DVT/PE
- **Family history of thrombosis***
- Positive factor V Leiden
- Positive prothrombin 20210A
- Elevated serum homocysteine
- Positive lupus anticoagulant
- Elevated anticardiolipin antibodies
- Heparin-induced thrombocytopenia (HIT)
- Other congenital or acquired thrombophilia If yes:

Type________________

***most frequently missed risk factor**

For Women Only (Each Represents 1 Point)

- Oral contraceptives or hormone replacement therapy
- Pregnancy or postpartum (<1 month)
- History of unexplained stillborn infant, recurrent spontaneous abortion (≥ 3), premature birth with toxemia or growth-restricted infant

Total Risk Factor Score ☐

Figure 1. The 2005 Caprini Risk Assessment Model. Reprinted from Disease-a-Month, 51, Caprini JA, Thrombosis Risk Assessment as a Guide to Quality Patient Care, 70-78., Copyright 2005, with permission from Elsevier.

Effectiveness of Chemical Thromboprophylaxis

The efficacy of chemical VTE prophylaxis has been widely reported in patients undergoing colectomy, [21] orthopedic hip surgery, [22] chemotherapy for pancreatic cancer, [23] ambulatory chemotherapy, [24] and medically ill patients. [25] In plastic and reconstructive surgery patients, a multicenter trial of 1,458 patients at moderate to high risk for VTE, defined by a Caprini score of ≥ 3, were treated only postoperatively with LMWH for the duration of their hospital stay. [26] This group was then compared against 1,876 historical control patients for the primary endpoint of symptomatic VTE reduction. [26] In patients with a Caprini score > 8, untreated patients developed symptomatic VTE at a rate over 8.5%. Comparatively, patients with a Caprini score > 8 who received LMWH prophylaxis developed VTE at a rate of 4%. When controlling for length of stay and Caprini score, LMWH significantly reduced the odds of VTE to 0.39.

Determination of the ideal pharmacologic anticoagulant for VTE prevention is an active area of research. In addition to UH and LMWH, a variety of direct thrombin and factor Xa inhibitors have been evaluated for VTE prophylaxis. A systematic review comparing LMWH to direct thrombin and factor Xa inhibitors suggested decreased VTE in fondaparinux and rivaroxaban treated patients, but also conferred greater risk of hemorrhage. [27] A multicenter retrospective cohort study of over 32,000 medical patients demonstrated equivalent efficacy and cost of UH and LMWH prophylaxis. [3] In a similarly large multicenter trial of over 24,000 bariatric surgery patients, LMWH was superior to UH in VTE prevention with no differences in hemorrhage. [28] Current society recommendations advocate the use of LMWH, and use of UH only when LMWH is contraindicated. As more data becomes available on direct thrombin and factor Xa inhibitors, guidelines may be updated to recommend their use as first line prophylaxis.

Risk of Hemorrhage

Risk of hemorrhage and return to the operating room is the most common reason cited by surgeons for non-adherence to ACCP guidelines. [11] There are mixed reports in the literature regarding the risk of hematoma with pharmaceutical VTE prophylaxis. In a longitudinal prospective trial of 425 patients who underwent modified radical mastectomy, simple mastectomy, and breast conserving surgery with level 1 and 2 axillary lymph node clearance, LMWH administration was associated with a 3-fold increase in risk for hematoma compared to thigh-long graduated compression stockings. [29] A longitudinal study of over 4,000 breast surgeries, ranging from breast biopsy to mastectomy to latissimus dorsi flap, comparing UH to LMWH for VTE prophylaxis, demonstrated LMWH was associated with a four-fold increase in relative risk of hemorrhage requiring surgical intervention compared to UH [30]. In contrast, a longitudinal study of 3,681 plastic and reconstructive surgery patients found that postoperative LMWH was not an independent predictor of re-operative hematoma. [31] Similarly, a systematic review of 33 randomized controlled clinical trials including over 33,800 general surgery patients demonstrated no significant difference in major bleeding and no difference in re-operative hemorrhage. [32] Given that the rate of re-operative hematoma formation ranges between 3-8% for breast surgery, [31,33] pharmaceutical thromboprophylaxis should be considered for moderate VTE risk patients with low bleeding risk and administered to all high and super-high VTE risk patients.

Risk factors

Risk factors associated with VTE in breast cancer patients have been investigated by Tran et al., using the American College of Surgeons National Surgical Quality Improvement Program (ACS-NSQIP) database. [1] In 49,028 mastectomy patients abstracted from the ACS-NSQIP database, 0.23% of patients developed VTE within 30 days of surgery. Inpatient status (OR = 3.75), BMI > 30 (OR = 1.91), central venous catheterization (OR = 2.67), and operative time > 3 hours (OR = 4.36) were all found to be independent risk factors of VTE. [1] Patient age, obesity and operative time are included within the Caprini RAM, however inpatient status and central venous catheterization are independently associated with significant VTE risk and should also be considered when determining if pharmaceutical VTE prophylaxis is indicated.

Approximately 70% of breast cancers are estrogen receptor positive, therefore the use of hormonal agents is widespread among breast cancer and mastectomy patients. Tamoxifen is a selective estrogen receptor modulator that has been used as an adjuvant therapeutic for over 30 years. Tamoxifen use has been shown to decrease anticoagulation factors including anti-thrombin III, protein C, and plasminogen activator inhibitor-1, as well as increase serum levels of prothrombotic factors VIII, IX, and von Willebrand factor. [34,35] This provides a potential pathway for the prothrombotic state of tamoxifen treated patients. Multiple studies from around the world have clearly demonstrated increased risk of VTE in women taking tamoxifen. [36] An Italian study of 5,408 hysterectomized women who were randomized to 5 years of tamoxifen or placebo demonstrated a VTE hazard ratio of 1.63 with tamoxifen use. [37] Similarly, in Scotland, a randomized study of 1,312 women who underwent mastectomy and were not treated with tamoxifen had a 60% reduced VTE risk compared to tamoxifen treated patients. [38] The increase in VTE risk appears to be concentrated at initiation of tamoxifen therapy, and longer-term use is associated with only incrementally increased cumulative risk of VTE. [39] At five years, the cumulative risk of VTE in tamoxifen treated patients ranges from 5-9%. [34,39] Many surgeons have developed their own algorithms for discontinuation of tamoxifen therapy in the perioperative period, but the effect on local recurrence, tumor free survival, and VTE risk are all unknown. One proposed algorithm which is based on VTE risk factors and tamoxifen pharmacokinetics recommends continuation of tamoxifen in the lowest risk patients, discontinuation of tamoxifen 3 weeks prior to surgery and resumption of dosing postoperatively in moderate risk patients, and discontinuation of tamoxifen 3 weeks before surgery and LMWH with graduated compression stockings until the patient is fully mobile in the highest risk patients. [40] With new data from the multinational ATLAS trial demonstrating decreased breast cancer recurrence, breast cancer mortality, and overall mortality with 10-year tamoxifen use compared to 5-year use, [41] the risk of VTE will continue to rise and the role of pharmaceutical VTE prophylaxis will become increasingly important.

Hormone receptor-negative breast cancer, select stage II and III, and all stage IV breast cancer patients are prescribed systemic chemotherapy, which may be administered as neoadjuvant or adjuvant therapy. Systemic chemotherapeutics are found to induce VTE through acute vessel damage, endothelial injury, and reduction in anticoagulation factors. [36] In a randomized phase III clinical trial of over 2,600 breast cancer patients stage I through IIIa, patients who underwent resection with adjuvant fluorouracil, doxorubicin, and cyclophosphamide developed VTE at a rate of 2.3% within 6 weeks after surgery compared to 0.8% rate of VTE in patients who underwent surgical resection alone. Additionally, patients who underwent mastectomy were 3.3 times more likely to develop VTE than patients who had local excision of the tumor. [42] A smaller trial of 134 breast cancer patients followed up to 12 months, found that 9.7% of patients receiving systemic chemotherapy developed VTE, which translated into a 28 day mortality rate of 15% after VTE diagnosis. [43] Depending on the duration of follow-up and systemic chemotherapeutic regimen, the reported rate of VTE in chemotherapy treated stage I and II breast cancer patients ranges from 0-13.6%. [36] With significantly increased risk and reported rates of VTE in breast cancer patients and mastectomy patients receiving systemic chemotherapy, physicians must seriously consider initiation and maintenance of pharmacological VTE prophylaxis in breast cancer patients.

VTE and Breast Reconstruction

Breast cancer patients requiring a mastectomy for their disease process may opt to undergo reconstruction. In fact, a review of the Surveillance,

Epidemiology, and End results (SEER) database from 1998-2002 revealed that 17% of women who underwent mastectomy also underwent immediate or delayed breast reconstruction and this number continues to rise. [44] The reconstruction can be performed either immediately after the mastectomy (i.e., in the same operation) or delayed to allow for future reconstruction. There are also several reconstructive options that can be performed depending on a variety of factors including the patient's body habitus. The different forms of reconstruction fit into two categories: (1) implant based reconstruction and (2) autologous tissue transfer. Autologous tissue transfer can be performed using transverse rectus abdominis musculocutaneous (TRAM) flaps, deep inferior epigastric perforator (DIEP) flaps, and latissimus dorsi flaps. TRAM and DIEP flaps can be further subdivided into pedicled and free flaps.

Table 2. Previous Studies Examining Rates of VTE in Patients Undergoing Breast Cancer Surgery and Reconstruction

Year	Author	Reconstruction Type	N	Number DVT (Rate)	Number PE (Rate)	VTE Rate
2007	Spear et al., [46]	Pedicle TRAM	200	1 (0.5%)	2(1.0%)	1.5%
2006	Mehrara et al., [47]	Free flap after mastectomy	952	9(0.95%)	0	0.95%
2006	Andtabaka et al., [5]	Breast cancer ± reconstruction	4416	3(0.07%)	4(0.09%)	0.16%
2005	Olsson et al., [48]	Delayed free TRAM	16	2(12.5%)	1(6.3%)	18.8%
2005	Wang et al., [49]	Pedicle TRAM	107	2(1.9%)	1(0.9%)	2.8%
2005	Gabbay et al., [50]	Pedicle midabdominal TRAM	18	0	0	0
2005	Spear et al., [51]	Pedicle TRAM ± XRT	150	1(0.7%)	1(0.7%)	1.3%
2005	Spear et al., [46]	Pedicle TRAM	200	1(0.5%)	2(1.0%)	1.5%
2004	Guerra et al., [52]	Bilateral DIEP	140	1(0.8%)	0	0.8%
2004	Hamdi et al., [53]	Bilateral perforator flaps	53	2(3.8%)	0	3.8%
1991	Arnez et al., [54]	Free TRAM	50	1(2.0%)	1(2.0%)	4.0%
1987	Hartrampf et al., [55]	Pedicle, delayed TRAM	300	0	2(0.67%)	0.67%

Adapted from Pannucci CJ, Chang EY, Wilkins EG. Venous Thromboembolic Disease in Autogenous Breast Reconstruction. *Annals of Plastic Surgery* 2009; 63 (1): 34-38 [45]

Studies have estimated a range of VTE incidence from 0-18.8% in patients undergoing breast cancer reconstruction. [45] There have been several small and large studies addressing the rates of VTE in patients undergoing chest wall reconstruction after breast surgery (Table 2).

These studies investigated a range of reconstructive surgeries from free flaps to pedicled TRAMs, with and without radiation. In 2005, Spear et al., examined the effect of radiation on pedicled TRAM flaps in breast reconstruction and identified 1 PE and 1 DVT in 150 patients, both of which occurred in post-TRAM patients who received radiation. [51] At a VTE incidence of 1.7%, statistical significance was not reached. [51] This paper also did not address if peri-operative prophylaxis was administered. Wang et al., investigated data in pedicled TRAM flap reconstructions and found 2 DVTs and 1 PE for an overall VTE incidence of 2.8% among 107 patients. [49] Of note, the two patients that were found to have a DVT were also morbidly obese. Again, no details were revealed about VTE prophylaxis in the study population. Mehrara et al., reviewed data from free flap reconstruction, the majority of which were TRAM flaps after a mastectomy, and found a VTE incidence rate as low as 0.95%. [47] Prophylaxis, again, was not clearly noted in these patients. While these studies targeted a specific type of reconstruction, the size of the study was moderate.

A larger study in 2006 by Andtabaka et al., studied 3898 patients who underwent 4,416 breast cancer operations and 18% of these patients also underwent immediate reconstruction with tissue expanders or flaps. [5] A total of 7 patients among the 3,898 developed a DVT or PE within 60 days after surgery. Since breast reconstructive procedures can often take longer than mastectomy portion of the operation a confounding variable may be overall operative time. The authors showed that mean operative time was 125 minutes (range of 9-585 minutes with a median time of 117 minutes) in the patients who did not undergo immediate reconstruction and a mean operative time of 466 minutes (range of 74-1,104 minutes with a median of 442 minutes) among those who did undergo immediate reconstruction. However, when studying the patients who developed a VTE, the mean operative time was 278 minutes, which was greater than the mean operative time of 186 minutes in all the breast surgery patients but was not statistically significant. Although these papers noted incidence of DVT and PE, the studies were not designed solely for that purpose, and as such, also did not clarify the prophylaxis regimen that patients received during the studies. While all of these studies shed light on the incidence and significance of VTE in breast reconstruction patients, they still do not target the appropriate regimen to prevent VTE in this population.

At the current time, there are no published guidelines for VTE prevention in breast cancer patients undergoing breast reconstruction; however, several studies have begun to address VTE prophylaxis in this patient population. Pannucci et al., published a retrospective review of 271 patients at the University of Michigan over a 10 year span who underwent autologous breast reconstruction with either a TRAM (free or pedicled), a DIEP, or a latissimus dorsi flap (immediate or delayed). [45] Only 4.4% of the study patients received preoperative pharmacologic prophylaxis and 11.8% received postoperative pharmacologic prophylaxis. [45] Of note, in the middle of the study (mid-2006), the hospital also changed its prophylaxis policy according to ACCP guidelines and provided postoperative pharmacologic prophylaxis to all their patients. All patients in this study had IPCs placed and started before anesthesia induction and throughout their hospital stay. A VTE incidence of 2.2% was found in this study, with one of the six cases occurring in a patient with known Factor V Leiden mutation. This study, being a retrospective analysis, may underestimate the actual incidence of VTE in this patient population as these were based on ultrasound studies obtained only in symptomatic patients.

In 2010, Disa et al., published a prospective cohort study on VTE following microsurgical breast reconstruction using LMWH. [56] A total of 225 consecutive women were enrolled, 75.1% of which had a breast cancer diagnosis. [56] These women underwent either a free TRAM flap, a free muscle-sparing TRAM flap, or a DIEP flap after therapeutic or prophylactic mastectomy. Of the women enrolled, 118 underwent bilateral lower extremity duplex ultrasound prior to discharge to assess for DVT and a retrospective cohort of 107 women who did not undergo ultrasound were used for comparison. [56] All patients were placed on triple thromboprophylaxis: postoperative dalteparin (LMWH), IPC before anesthesia induction, and early ambulation in accordance with the 2008 ACCP guidelines. This study found an objective incidence of asymptomatic distal lower extremity DVT of 3.4% within 5 days of breast reconstruction with an abdominal free flap for patients on triple thromboprophylactic regimen. [56] These results show that using triple therapy thromboprophylaxis is effective in this population of patients and that asymptomatic and subclinical VTE is common among breast reconstruction patients. This study also calls into question whether or not patients who are at high risk for a VTE predicted by the Caprini model should be screened via ultrasound duplex for a DVT regardless of symptoms.

While Disa et al., show that triple therapy thromboprophylaxis is effective, the concern in post-surgical plastic reconstruction patients is bleeding and hematoma risk. Kim et al., conducted a prospective study over a six-year period on 650 patients that underwent immediate breast reconstruction using a TRAM flap. [57] The first 450 patients did not receive pharmacologic prophylaxis, whereas the next 200 patients, after mid 2006, received routine LMWH for 7 days immediately following surgery. The incidence of symptomatic pulmonary thromboembolism did not differ significantly between the two groups; however, the incidence of asymptomatic pulmonary thromboembolism was significantly higher in the group that did not receive any prophylaxis ($p=0.009$). [57] Interestingly, there was no significant difference in the incidence of hematoma, seroma, or transfusion between the two groups. This led to the conclusion that not only was LMWH effective against preventing pulmonary thromboembolism, but it also did not present any increased bleeding related complication.

Using the ACS-NSQIP database, Tran et al., sought to specifically identify the risk factors associated with VTE in mastectomy patients. They identified 114 cases of VTE in 49,028 cases that underwent mastectomy and further analyzed for risk factors. [1] Immediate reconstruction was found to be one of four intraoperative statistically significant risk factors for VTE in these patients ($p<0.001$). Of the 9,571 patients who underwent immediate reconstruction, 50 of them were found to have a VTE. This constitutes 44% of all the patients observed to have a VTE in this study. After multivariable logistic regression analysis to derive adjusted risk for VTE in this population, Tran et al., found immediate reconstruction to not be statistically significant as a risk factor. [1] Although not significant alone after risk adjustment, immediate reconstruction may still contribute to the outcome. Autologous flaps require prolonged operative time, and operative time over 3 hours was also found to be an independent risk factor of VTE after risk adjustment.

Conclusion

The incidence of VTE in breast cancer patients undergoing mastectomy with or without reconstruction is considerable. This incidence combined with the morbidity and mortality associated with VTE in this patient population, makes this disease an important area of continued research. Studies have been published to identify the independent risk factors and quantify the risks and benefits of pharmacologic and mechanical prophylaxis. Further studies that address VTE and prophylaxis in the several different breast reconstruction options will improve the understanding of VTE in this population. As data accumulates, we endorse formal establishment of guidelines for VTE prophylaxis in breast cancer patients undergoing mastectomy with or without breast reconstruction.

References

[1] Tran BH, Nguyen TJ, Hwang BH, et al., Risk factors associated with venous thromboembolism in 49,028 mastectomy patients. *Breast.* 2013;22(4):444–8.

[2] U.S. Cancer Statistics Working Group. *United States Cancer Statistics: 1999–2010 Incidence and Mortality Web-based Report.* Atlanta: U.S. Department of Health and Human Services, Centers for Disease Control and Prevention and National Cancer Institute; 2013. Available at: www.cdc.gov/uscs.

[3] Rothberg MB, Pekow PS, Lahti M, Lindenauer PK. Comparative effectiveness of low-molecular-weight heparin versus unfractionated heparin for thromboembolism prophylaxis for medical patients. *J. Hosp. Med.* 7(6):457–63.

[4] Colzani E, Liljegren A, Johansson ALV, et al., Prognosis of patients with breast cancer: Causes of death and effects of time since diagnosis, age, and tumor characteristics. *J. Clin. Oncol.* 2011;29:4014-21.

[5] Andtbacka RHI, Babiera G, Singletary SE, et al., Incidence and prevention of venous thromboembolism in patients undergoing breast cancer surgery and treated according to clinical pathways. *Ann. Surg.* 2006;243(1):96–101.

[6] American Society of Breast Surgeons. Position statement on venous thromoembolism prophylaxis for patients undergoing breast operations. 2011.

[7] Auer RAC, Scheer AS, McSparron JI, et al., Postoperative Venous Thromboembolism Predicts Survival in Cancer Patients. *Ann. Surg.* 2012;255(5):963–970.

[8] Wedgwood KR, Benson EA. Non-tumour morbidity and mortality after modified radical mastectomy. *Ann. R. Coll. Surg. Engl.* 1992;74(5):314–7.

[9] Chew HK, Wun T, Harvey DJ, Zhou H, White RH. Incidence of venous thromboembolism and the impact on survival in breast cancer patients. *J. Clin. Oncol.* 2007;25(1):70–6.

[10] Gould MK, Garcia DA, Wren SM, et al., Prevention of VTE in nonorthopedic surgical patients: antithrombotic therapy and prevention of thrombosis, 9th ed: American College of Chest Physicians evidence-based clinical practice guidelines. *Chest.* 2012;141(2)(suppl):e227S-e277S.

[11] Pannucci CJ, Oppenheimer AJ, Wilkins EG. Practice patterns in venous thromboembolism prophylaxis: a survey of 606 reconstructive breast surgeons. *Ann. Plast. Surg.* 2010;64(6):732–7.

[12] Caprini JA, Arcelus JI, Hasty JH, Tamhane AC, Fabrega F. Clinical assessment of venous thromboembolic risk in surgical patients. *Semin. Thromb. Hemost.* 1991;17 Suppl 3:304–12.

[13] Pannucci CJ, Barta RJ, Portschy PR, et al., Assessment of postoperative venous thromboembolism risk in plastic surgery patients using the 2005 and 2010 Caprini Risk score. *Plast. Reconstr. Surg.* 2012;130(2):343–53.

[14] Yarlagadda BB, Brook CD, Stein DJ, Jalisi S. Venous thromboembolism in otolaryngology surgical inpatients receiving chemoprophylaxis. *Head Neck.* 2013.

[15] Bahl V, Hu HM, Henke PK, Wakefield TW, Campbell DA, Caprini JA. A validation study of a retrospective venous thromboembolism risk scoring method. *Ann. Surg.* 2010;251(2):344–50.

[16] Gould MK, Garcia DA, Wren SM, et al., Prevention of VTE in nonorthopedic surgical patients: Antithrombotic Therapy and Prevention of Thrombosis, 9th ed: American College of Chest Physicians Evidence-Based Clinical Practice Guidelines. *Chest.* 2012;141(2 Suppl):e227S–77S.

[17] Caprini JA. Thrombosis risk assessment as a guide to quality patient care. *Dis. Mon.* 51(2-3):70–8.

[18] Kakkos SK, Caprini JA, Geroulakos G, Nicolaides AN, Stansby GP, Reddy DJ. Combined intermittent pneumatic leg compression and pharmacological prophylaxis for prevention of venous thromboembolism in high-risk patients. *Cochrane database Syst. Rev.* 2008;(4):CD005258.

[19] Sobieraj DM, Coleman CI, Tongbram V, et al., Comparative effectiveness of combined pharmacologic and mechanical thromboprophylaxis versus either method alone in major orthopedic surgery: a systematic review and meta-analysis. *Pharmacotherapy.* 2013;33(3):275–83.

[20] Pannucci CJ, Bailey SH, Dreszer G, et al., Validation of the Caprini risk assessment model in plastic and reconstructive surgery patients. *J. Am. Coll. Surg.* 2011;212(1):105–12.

[21] Henke PK, Arya S, Pannucci C, et al., Procedure-specific venous thromboembolism prophylaxis: a paradigm from colectomy surgery. *Surgery.* 2012;152(4):528–34; discussion 534–6.

[22] Fisher WD, Agnelli G, George DJ, et al., Extended venous thromboembolism prophylaxis in patients undergoing hip fracture surgery - the SAVE-HIP3 study. *Bone Joint J.* 2013;95-B(4):459–66.

[23] Maraveyas A, Waters J, Roy R, et al., Gemcitabine versus gemcitabine plus dalteparin thromboprophylaxis in pancreatic cancer. *Eur. J. Cancer.* 2012;48(9):1283–92.

[24] Di Nisio M, Porreca E, Ferrante N, Otten H-M, Cuccurullo F, Rutjes AWS. Primary prophylaxis for venous thromboembolism in ambulatory cancer patients receiving chemotherapy. *Cochrane database Syst. Rev.* 2012;2:CD008500.

[25] Baser O, Liu X, Phatak H, et al., Venous thromboembolism prophylaxis and clinical consequences in medically ill patients. *Am. J. Ther.* 20(2):132–42.

[26] Pannucci CJ, Dreszer G, Wachtman CF, et al., Postoperative enoxaparin prevents symptomatic venous thromboembolism in high-risk plastic surgery patients. *Plast. Reconstr. Surg.* 2011;128(5):1093–103.

[27] Yoshida R de A, Yoshida WB, Maffei FH de A, El Dib R, Nunes R, Rollo HA. Systematic review of randomized controlled trials of new anticoagulants for venous thromboembolism prophylaxis in major orthopedic surgeries, compared with enoxaparin. *Ann. Vasc. Surg.* 2013;27(3):355–69.

[28] Birkmeyer NJO, Finks JF, Carlin AM, et al., Comparative effectiveness of unfractionated and low-molecular-weight heparin for prevention of venous thromboembolism following bariatric surgery. *Arch. Surg.* 2012;147(11):994–8.

[29] Friis E, Hørby J, Sørensen LT, et al., Thromboembolic prophylaxis as a risk factor for postoperative complications after breast cancer surgery. *World J. Surg.* 2004;28(6):540–3.

[30] Hardy RG, Williams L, Dixon JM. Use of enoxaparin results in more haemorrhagic complications after breast surgery than unfractionated heparin. *Br. J. Surg.* 2008;95(7):834–6.

[31] Pannucci CJ, Wachtman CF, Dreszer G, et al., The effect of postoperative enoxaparin on risk for reoperative hematoma. *Plast. Reconstr. Surg.* 2012;129(1):160–8.

[32] Leonardi MJ, McGory ML, Ko CY. The rate of bleeding complications after pharmacologic deep venous thrombosis prophylaxis: a systematic review of 33 randomized controlled trials. *Arch. Surg.* 2006;141(8):790–7; discussion 797–9.

[33] Cunningham BL, Gear AJL, Kerrigan CL, Collins ED. Analysis of breast reduction complications derived from the BRAVO study. *Plast. Reconstr. Surg.* 2005;115(6):1597–604.

[34] Pemberton KD, Melissari E, Kakkar V V. The influence of tamoxifen in vivo on the main natural anticoagulants and fibrinolysis. *Blood Coagul. Fibrinolysis.* 1993;4(6):935–42.

[35] Cosman F, Baz-Hecht M, Cushman M, et al., Short-term effects of estrogen, tamoxifen and raloxifene on hemostasis: a randomized-controlled study and review of the literature. *Thromb. Res.* 2005;116(1):1–13.

[36] Biron-Andréani C, Elalamy I, Mandalà M, Tondini C. Adjuvant therapy in breast cancer and venous thromboembolism. *Thromb. Res.* 2012;130:S66–S70.

[37] Decensi A, Maisonneuve P, Rotmensz N, et al., Effect of tamoxifen on venous thromboembolic events in a breast cancer prevention trial. *Circulation.* 2005;111(5):650–6.

[38] McDonald CC, Alexander FE, Whyte BW, Forrest AP, Stewart HJ. Cardiac and vascular morbidity in women receiving adjuvant tamoxifen for breast cancer in a randomised trial. The Scottish Cancer Trials Breast Group. *BMJ.* 1995;311(7011):977–80.

[39] Onitilo AA, Doi SAR, Engel JM, Glurich I, Johnson J, Berg R. Clustering of venous thrombosis events at the start of tamoxifen therapy in breast cancer: A population-based experience. *Thromb. Res.* 2012;130(1):27–31.

[40] Hussain T, Kneeshaw PJ. Stopping tamoxifen peri-operatively for VTE risk reduction: A proposed management algorithm. *Int. J. Surg.* 2012;10(6):313–316.

[41] Davies C, Pan H, Godwin J, et al., Long-term effects of continuing adjuvant tamoxifen to 10 years versus stopping at 5 years after diagnosis of oestrogen receptor-positive breast cancer: ATLAS, a randomised trial. *Lancet.* 2013;381(9869):805–16.

[42] Clahsen PC, van de Velde CJ, Julien JP, Floiras JL, Mignolet FY. Thromboembolic complications after perioperative chemotherapy in women with early breast cancer: a European Organization for Research and Treatment of Cancer Breast Cancer Cooperative Group study. *J. Clin. Oncol.* 1994;12(6):1266–71.

[43] Kirwan CC, McDowell G, McCollum CN, Byrne GJ. Incidence of venous thromboembolism during chemotherapy for breast cancer: impact on cancer outcome. *Anticancer Res.* 2011;31(6):2383–8.

[44] Agarwal, S., Liu, J. H., Crisera, C. A., Buys, S. and Agarwal, J. P. (2010), Survival in Breast Cancer Patients Undergoing Immediate Breast Reconstruction. *Breast*, 16: 503–509.

[45] Pannucci CJ, Chang EY, Wilkins EG. Venous Thromboembolic Disease in Autogenous Breast Reconstruction. *Annals of Plastic Surgery* 2009; 63 (1): 34-38.

[46] Spear SL, Ducic I, Cuoco F, et al., Effect of obesity on flap and donor-site complications in pedicled TRAM flap breast reconstruction. *Plast. Reconstr. Surg*. 2007;119:788–795.

[47] Mehrara BJ, Santoro TD, Arcilla E, et al., Complications after microvascular breast reconstruction: experience with 1195 flaps. *Plast. Reconstr. Surg*. 2006; 118: 1100–1109; discussion 1110–1111.

[48] Olsson EH, Tukiainen E. Three-year evaluation of late breast reconstruction with a free transverse rectus abdominis musculocutaneous flap in a county hospital in Sweden: a retrospective study. *Scand J Plast. Reconstr. Surg Hand Surg*. 2005;39:33–38.

[49] Wang HT, Hartzell T, Olbrich KC, et al., Delay of transverse rectus abdominis myocutaneous flap reconstruction improves flap reliability in the obese patient. *Plast. Reconstr. Surg*. 2005; 116: 613–618; discussion 619–620.

[50] Gabbay JS, Eby JB, Kulber DA. The midabdominal TRAM flap for breast reconstruction in morbidly obese patients. *Plast. Reconstr. Surg*. 2005;115: 764 –770.

[51] Spear SL, Ducic I, Low M, et al., The effect of radiation on pedicled TRAM flap breast reconstruction: outcomes and implications. *Plast. Reconstr. Surg*. 2005; 115: 84 –95.

[52] Guerra AB, Soueid N, Metzinger SE, et al., Simultaneous bilateral breast reconstruction with superior gluteal artery perforator (SGAP) flaps. *Ann. Plast. Surg*. 2004;53:305–310.

[53] Hamdi M, Blondeel P, Van Landuyt K, et al., Bilateral autogenous breast reconstruction using perforator free flaps: a single center's experience. *Plast. Reconstr. Surg*. 2004;114:83–89; discussion 90–92.

[54] Arnez ZM, Bajec J, Bardsley AF, et al., Experience with 50 free TRAM flap breast reconstructions. *Plast. Reconstr. Surg*. 1991;87:470 – 478; discussion 479 – 482.

[55] Hartrampf CR. Breast reconstruction with a transverse abdominal island flap. *Persp. Plast. Surg*. 1987;1:123–135.

[56] Lemain V, McCarthy C, Kaplan K, et al., Venous thromboembolism following microsurgical breast reconstruction: an objective analysis in 225 consecutive patients using low-molecular-weight heparin prophylaxis. *Plast. Reconstr. Surg*. 2010; 127(4): 1399-1406.

[57] Kim EK, Eom JS, Ahn SH, et al., The efficacy of prophylactic low-molecular-weight heparin to prevent pulmonary thromboembolism in immediate breast reconstruction using the TRAM flap. *Plast. Reconstr. Surg*. 2008; 123(1): 9-12.

In: Venous Thrombosis
Editor: Caroline H. Gutmann
ISBN: 978-1-63117-293-9

Chapter 2

Calf Vein Thrombosis

Indraneil Mukherjee, M.D., Khanjan H. Nagarsheth, M.D. and Kuldeep Singh, M.D.
Staten Island University Hospital,
Division of Vascular Surgery, Staten Island, NY, US

Abstract

The clinical significance of isolated calf vein thrombosis (ICVT) is controversial. It has not been adequately studied and its diagnostic and management guidelines are not universally similar. The majority of ICVTs are asymptomatic, diagnosed on screening ultrasound duplex sonography and do not propagate above the knee. A smaller portion of ICVTs are symptomatic and may propagate this subgroup can cause significant morbidity and even mortality. Management of ICVT differs among physicians and institutions. Some therapeutically anticoagulate, whereas some advise chemical and/or mechanical prophylaxis. Some physicians advise close surveillance with repetitive duplex scanning. For patients that are at high risk for clot propagation short term theoretic anticoagulation is recommended.

Keywords: Calf deep thrombosis, anticoagulation, pulmonary embolism

Introduction

Isolated Calf Vein Thrombosis (ICVT) is often a clinical conundrum as management guidelines vary among institutions and physicians. Its clinical relevance and treatment remains controversial because the natural history is largely unknown. The majority of ICVTs are asymptomatic, diagnosed on screening ultrasound duplex sonography and do not propagate above the knee. A small proportion of ICVTs are symptomatic, actually propagate and would need interventions to prevent further clot extension or pulmonary embolisms (PE). This group is concerning because calf vein thrombosis may be the starting point for deep vein thrombosis (DVT) of the lower extremity.

Anatomy

Isolated calf vein thrombosis is thrombosis involving the veins of the calf that does not extend into the popliteal vein. The calf veins include three paired veins that course along with the arteries of lower extremity. These include the posterior tibial, peroneal, and anterior tibial as well as two unpaired muscular veins, the soleal and gastrocnemius. The peroneal veins are located medially to the fibula; the posterior tibial veins are dorsal to the tibia, while the anterior tibial veins cross the interosseous membrane in the anterior compartment. [1] Usually the most common veins involved are the peroneal veins and posterior tibial [2-4]. The ICVTs are sometimes further divided into isolated calf muscle vein thrombosis (ICMVT) for a thrombosis confined to the soleus and gastrocnemius veins while deep calf vein thrombosis (DCVT) is reserved for a thrombosis present in the anterior tibial, posterior tibial and peroneal veins. [1]

Epidemiology

Rates of ICVT vary greatly among population and studies. The prevalence of ICVT ranges from about 7 to 11% in suspected PE, and 4 to 15% in cases of suspected DVT [1]. The prevalence of this disease is between 5% and 33% of all DVT cases detected by ultrasound [5]. In patients with PE, the incidence of proximal and distal thrombosis is 50% and 20%, respectively [6].

Risk Factors

The risk factors of ICVT were initially thought to be similar to DVT and PE. Newer studies interject that risk for developing ICVT may be different from risk factors involved in proximal DVT and PE. A prospective study from the RIETE registry [7], involving 11,086 patients revealed that recent travel, hospitalization, recent surgery and the presence of varicosities independently increased the risk of ICVTs, while the presence of proximal DVT was higher in peri-partum women, in elderly patients (≥75 years), in patients with cancer, recent major bleeding or a previous history of venous thromboembolism (VTE). Interestingly, the presence of inherited thrombophilic disorder had no effect on the prevalence of ICVT [7, 8].

Natural History

Isolated calf vein thrombosis can vary in symptomatology. The asymptomatic ICVTs usually involve smaller segments and rarely have long term consequences. They may propagate to proximal veins, embolize, lyse completely, or recanalize. As these rarely propagate and occlude the proximal veins post-thrombotic syndrome is not a usually seen.

One hypothesis proposes that DVTs actually start in the calf veins and then propagate to the proximal veins [9, 10], even though their risk factors may be different [7]. Clinically, the critical question lies in the rate of proximal propagation of these ICVTs. Predicting which ICVTs will propagate and thus need treatment is an ongoing debate. The natural history of ICVTs is different in different cases, based on the patient's risk factors [7]. The risk factors involved in ICVTs propogating are similar to proximal DVT or PE. Propagation rates reported in the literature, usually range from 4% to 34% in patients with symptomatic and asymptomatic calf DVT [2, 11-14]. Venous thromboembolism in patients with calf DVT ranges from 0% to 33%. [4] We know that ICVTs are at lower risk of recurrence and morbidity than bilateral ICVT [7, 15-17].

The CALTHRO study [18] suggests that proximal extension within 1 week occurs in 3% patients while more than 90% have complete resolution without any systemic anticoagulant therapy. Some literature states that ICMVT propagate less frequently than DCVT [19, 20].

Masuda [2] found complete lysis of in 88% of ICVTs studied at 90 days and 100% in 1 year. But 5% of the patients had persistent symptoms like hyperpigmentation and varicose veins at 3 years. These chronic symptoms constitute the post-thrombotic syndrome. This syndrome is rare in ICVTs and if they present with increased venous pressure they likely need obliteration or obstruction of the larger proximal veins. This syndrome was reported to have an incidence of 4% by Hirsch at collegeaus [21].

Diagnosis

The gold standard method of diagnosis for venous thrombosis is phlebography. Phlebography is technically challenging, invasive, and also a very expensive modality with only a few added advantages over non invasive techniques. Along with being invasive it has a significantly higher complication rate. The complications could be related to the venous access with hemorrhage and thrombosis of the accessed vein, or could be associated with valvular and intimal injury secondary to manipulations. It also may be contraindicated in patients with renal insufficiency or hypersensitivity to iodinated contrast mediums. It also has considerable intraobserver and interobserver variation with up to 20% of phlebographs having inadequate visualization [22]. Thus today the diagnostic modality of choice is duplex ultrasound (DUS).

The DUS has minimal associated complications and a much lower cost when compared to phlebography. Duplex ultrasound is readily available in most hospital and because it is portable, DUS has a higher outreach compared to phlebography, which is now used only for operative cases and rarely for diagnostic purpose. The accuracy of the DUS is dependant of the institution's examination protocol and the skills of the diagnostician and the reviewer of the images.

In an established center with experience, DUS results are similar to phlebography [23]. Its accuracy is as high as 94% [3]. Its sensitivity for symptomatic distal vein thrombosis is between 73% and 93% [24]. A metanalysis of 34 studies comparing DUS with phlebography for ICVTs in symptomatic patients found a specificity of 96.0% [22]. Poor blood flow can increase the echogenicity and cause false positive results. [25]

On the DUS venous thrombosis is diagnosed when an enlarged non-compressible vein is visualized. Color flow doppler helps to evaluate complete or incomplete thrombosis of the vessel. On visualization of the thrombus bidirectional evaluation is performed in multiple planes to see the entire thrombus. There will be a lack of flow augmentation on DUS.

The DUS is performed for two indications. As a screening test, it is done bilaterally and all the veins are examined in the B mode ultrasound for non-compressibility of the segment. The color flow doppler is used to visualize flow and echo duplex used to see lack of flow augmentation. When looking for ICVTs it is done from the knees down to the ankles along the venous anatomy which closely follows the arterial anatomy and also looks for deep muscular veins. For symptomatic patients all the same modalities should be used on the affected limb. As peroneal, posterior tibial, and gastrocnemius veins are the most commonly involved veins, [2] they should be actively identified for both screening and diagnostic DUS.

In most patients, especially high risk patients, maneuvers to distend the veins like hanging the leg in a dependant position or standing should be attempted to avoid false negative results.

The specificity of ultrasound in the detection of asymptomatic calf vein thrombosis is less than for symptomatic DVT [26, 27]. Isolated calf vein thrombosis accounts for up to 60% of all DVTs found on DUS. The DUS's accuracy to find ICVTs are much lower than diagnosing proximal DVTs [28]. Some feel phlebography is warranted in cases where DUS is nondiagnostic or discordant [29]. Many authors are proponent of serial DUS along with other clinical and laboratory assessments [30-33]. Using the pre test probability based algorithms set forth by Wells and colleagues [32, 33] allows patient stratification into low, moderate and high probability of DVT. Patients with moderate to high probability should have a repeat DUS after 7 to 14 days to assess for propagation of undetected ICVTs. Although these protocols for surveillance DUS are not standardized, they are advocated by some researchers. [34]

The American College of Chest Physicians (ACCP) Evidence-Based Clinical Practice Guidelines does not recommend screening DUS following major orthopedic surgery, trauma or acutely ill patients [26, 27, 35, 36]. They do recommend DUS screening in patients who are at high risk for VTE and in those who have received suboptimal or no prophylaxis [26]. Duplex ultrasound as a screening tool for distal deep vein thrombosis is not beneficial after major orthopedic surgery and was shown by a randomized controlled trial [37].

Deep venous thrombosis is common in critically ill trauma patients, regardless of injury pattern, risk factors, or prophylaxis and the ACCP may have underestimated DVT rates by not investigating ICVTs. Some reports show that up to 60% of DVTs identified in trauma patients are ICVTs [38].

Computed tomography (CT) venogram involves injection of contrast into a peripheral vein followed by scanning timed to opacify the veins of the lower extremity. It has the same drawbacks of venography except complication of cannulation of a leg vein. The advantage is that it can be added to CT pulmonary angiography thus imaging for suspected both sides of VTE. Magnetic resonance imaging (MRI) can also be used to visualize the veins of the leg. MRI can directly identify the thrombus and the surrounding inflammation. Neither of these options are not used frequently for the diagnosis of DVT.

Antithrombotic Therapy and Prevention of Thrombosis's 9th edition by the American College of Chest Physicians [22] suggest that clinical assessment of pretest probability of DVT, rather than performing the same tests in all patients, should guide the diagnostic process for a first lower extremity DVT. In patients with a low pretest probability for lower extremity DVT, they recommend initial testing with D-dimer or DUS of the proximal veins. In patients with moderate pretest probability, they recommend initial testing with a D-dimer or DUS. In patients with a high pretest probability, the recommendation is DUS.

Management

The Management of ICVTs is controversial and variable among experts. It ranges from routine anticoagulation enterally or parentally to a variable regiment of surveillence studies and observation.

Despite the best guidelines and recommendations [26, 27], it is impossible to prevent ICVT in the high risk group. Mechanical and chemical thromboprophylaxis has been the major modalities in the preventing ICVTs. Mechanical thromboprophylaxis modalities have greater effect in reducing ICVTs than proximal DVT [26]. Chemical thromboprophylaxis needs to be used cautiously as possible bleeding complications may be higher especially in the high risk population.

The need to anticoagulate symptomatic ICVTs were established in 1985 by Lagerstedt and colleagues [14]. In a randomized trial they documented 29% of patients at 3 month and 32% of patients at 1 year to have recurrence or extension of their DVT when not treated with anticoagulation. The treatment arm had less than 4% extension or recurrence. The use of chemical thrombolytics has been considered for a long time. In 1986 low-dose streptokinase was used and it did show benefit but bleeding complications precluded it widespread use [39]. Thus the use of chemical thrombolytics was used only in extensive and symptomatic DVTs and anticoagulation remained the main stay of treatment.

In the DOTAVK study [16] the recurrence rate was found to be lower for patients with ICVTs (2.6%) than it was for those with proximal DVT or PE (8.4%). The study also showed equivalence between the treating ICVTS with anticoagulation for 6 or 12 weeks without a significant increase in bleeding complications. The TICT study [40] found that patients who were treated with a full dose of Low Molecular weight Heparin (LMWH) anticoagulation for 1 week followed by 3 weeks of half dose of LMWH showed reduced rates of propagation of proximal DVT and ICVT with rates of 2.9 and 1.1%, respectively.

As the need for anticoagulation was evident the modality of anticoagulation has evolved over a period of time. In 1986 continuous intravenous heparin proved better than intermittent subcutaneous heparin in the treatment of proximal-vein thrombosis, with recurrence of 5.2% compared to 19.3 % [41]. Hommes [42] showed that intermittent subcubaneous heparin was not only as safe but even more effective in treating DVTs. With the advent of low-molecular-weight heparin its subcutaneous cutaneous use was favored over intravenous unfractionated heparin in proximal DVTs [43]. This view has been reinforced by multiple authors [44-46]. LMWH was shown to decreases proximal DVT and also ICVTs following total knee arthroplasty [47].

With the advent of enteral Factor Xa inhibitors, there are alternatives to LMWH for prophylaxis and therapy. They may be used as a first line of prophylaxis or therapy instead of heparinoids. Fondaparinux one of the initial modalities proven and later approved to be useful for treatment of VTEs was also shown to have higher efficacy in prophylaxis as well [48, 49]. Its use in high-risk abdominal surgery was comparable to LMWH [50, 51]. Fondaparinux works by antithrombin III (ATIII)-mediated selective inhibition of Factor Xa. The newer indirect factor Xa inhibitors, idraparinux, idrabiotaparinux, and SR123781A, are second and third generation variants of fondaparinux [52] In the Van Gogh [53] trial, patients with DVT were given weekly subcutaneous Idraparinux for 3 or 6 months and were found to have an efficacy similar to that of heparin plus warfarin. Idrabiotaparinux has similar properties of Idraparinux with possibly less bleeding complications [54]. This medication has the added benefit of being reversible [55].

The newest generation of oral anticoagulants is the direct Factor Xa inhibitors like Rivaroxaban, Dabigatran, or Apixaban. Though these agents are felt to be efficacious, they are also concerning due to a lack of reversibility. They are generally associated with higher bleeding complications [56, 57]. They were found to be non-inferior to LMWH, especially in high risk patients [58-62].

Initially proven by McKenna [63] in 1980s, aspirin prevents VTE. The Antiplatelet Trialists' Collaboration [64] and PEP Trial [65] in 2000 started that Aspirin and anti-platelet drugs prevent venous thrombosis and PE. It is though inferior to modalities like complete anticoagulation [66] or the use of chemoprophylaxis [67].

Intermittent pneumatic compression (IPC) of the foot and calf improves the outcome of catheter-directed thrombolysis using low-dose urokinase in patients with acute proximal venous thrombosis of the leg [68]. Calf and thigh IPCs are better than IPCs of the feet in preventing DVT [69]. In a prospective randomized trial of 290 patients IPCs of the foot were proven to be better than LMWH for the prevention of DVT after orthopedic surgery [70]. Two large studies, one a large metanalysis [71] and another a systemic review [72] showed that IPC reduced the risk of DVT including asymptomatic DVT and ICVT by as much as by 60%. This data can be safely extrapolated to state that IPCs can be used as therapeutic as well as preventive for ICVTs.

The CLOTS (Clots in Legs Or sTockings after Stroke) Trial that compared Thigh-length versus below-knee graduated compression stockings (GCS) for deep venous thrombosis prophylaxis showed a reduction in the proximal DVT but not ICVT [73]. Therefore the GCS can have a prophylactic effect in high risk patients when chemical prophylaxis is not feasible.

The Antithrombotic Therapy and Prevention of Thrombosis's 9th edition by the American College of Chest Physicians [27] states that patients with acute ICVT with severe symptoms or risk factors for extension should be initially anticoagulated. In cases where anticoagulation was started they recommend to continue as per protocols for management of proximal DVT. In cases that were managed with serial DUS they do not recommend anticoagulation if the thrombus does not extend, but if extension occurs, anticoagulation should be initiated. Cases at high risk for bleeding are more likely to benefit from serial DUS whereas patients who have a low risk of bleeding and cannot have serial DUS may benefit from anticoagulation.

References

[1] Palareti G, Schellong S. Isolated distal deep vein thrombosis: What we know and what we are doing. *Journal of Thrombosis and Haemostasis.* 2012;10(1):11-9.

[2] Masuda EM, Kessler DM, Kistner RL, Eklof B, Sato DT, DePalma R, et al. The natural history of calf vein thrombosis: Lysis of thrombi and development of reflux. *Journal of Vascular Surgery.* 1998;28(1):67-74.

[3] Mattos MA, Melendres G, Sumner DS, Hood DB, Barkmeier LD, Hodgson KJ, et al. Prevalence and distribution of calf vein thrombosis in patients with symptomatic deep venous thrombosis: A color-flow duplex study. *Journal of Vascular Surgery.* 1996;24(5):738-44.

[4] Labropoulos N, Webb KM, Kang SS, Mansour MA, Filliung DR, Size GP, et al. Patterns and distribution of isolated calf deep vein thrombosis. *Journal of Vascular Surgery.* 1999;30(5):787-93.

[5] Antignani PL, Aluigi L. The calf vein thrombosis. *Reviews in Vascular Medicine.* 2013;1(1):1-4.

[6] Seinturier C, Bosson JL, Colonna M, Imbert B, Carpentier PH. Site and clinical outcome of deep vein thrombosis of the lower limbs: An epidemiological study. *Journal of Thrombosis and Haemostasis.* 2005;3(7):1362-7.

[7] Galanaud JP, Quenet S, Rivron-Guillot K, Quere I, Sanchez Muñoz-Torrero JF, Tolosa C, et al. Comparison of the clinical history of symptomatic isolated distal deep-vein thrombosis vs. proximal deep vein thrombosis in 11086 patients. *Journal of Thrombosis and Haemostasis.* 2009;7(12):2028-34.

[8] Kovac M, Mitic G, Mikovic Z, Antonijevic N, Djordjevic V, Mikovic D, et al. Type and location of venous thromboembolism in carriers of Factor V Leiden or prothrombin G20210A mutation versus patients with no mutation. *Clin. Appl. Thromb. Hemost.* 2010;16(1):66-70.

[9] Nicolaides AN, Kakkar VV, Field ES, Renney JT. The origin of deep vein thrombosis: a venographic study. *Br. J. Radiol.* 1971;44(525):653-63.

[10] Rollins DL, Semrow CM, Friedell ML, Lloyd WE, Buchbinder D. Origin of deep vein thrombi in an ambulatory population. *Am. J. Surg.* 1988;156(2):122-5.

[11] Kakkar VV, Howe CT, Flanc C, Clarke MB. Natural history of postoperative deep-vein thrombosis. *Lancet.* 1969;2(7614):230-2.

[12] Lohr JM, Kerr TM, Lutter KS, Cranley RD, Spirtoff K, Cranley JJ. Lower extremity calf thrombosis: to treat or not to treat? *J. Vasc. Surg.* 1991;14(5):618-23.

[13] Meissner MH, Caps MT, Bergelin RO, Manzo RA, Strandness DE, Jr. Early outcome after isolated calf vein thrombosis. *J. Vasc. Surg.* 1997;26(5):749-56.

[14] Lagerstedt CI, Olsson CG, Fagher BO, Oqvist BW, Albrechtsson U. Need for long-term anticoagulant treatment in symptomatic calf-vein thrombosis. *Lancet.* 1985;2(8454):515-8.

[15] Schulman S, Rhedin AS, Lindmarker P, Carlsson A, Lärfars G, Nicol P, et al. A comparison of six weeks with six months of oral anticoagulant therapy after a first episode of venous thromboembolism. *New England Journal of Medicine.* 1995;332(25):1661-5.

[16] Pinede L, Ninet J, Duhaut P, Chabaud S, Demolombe-Rague S, Durieu I, et al. Comparison of 3 and 6 months of oral anticoagulant therapy after a first episode of proximal deep vein thrombosis or pulmonary embolism and comparison of 6 and 12 weeks of therapy after isolated calf deep vein thrombosis. *Circulation.* 2001;103(20):2453-60.

[17] Eichinger S, Heinze G, Jandeck LM, Kyrle PA. Risk assessment of recurrence in patients with unprovoked deep vein thrombosis or pulmonary embolism: The vienna prediction model. *Circulation.* 2010;121(14):1630-6.

[18] Palareti G, Cosmi B, Lessiani G, Rodorigo G, Guazzaloca G, Brusi C, et al. *Thrombosis and Haemostasis.* 2010;104(5):1063-70.

[19] Macdonald PS, Kahn SR, Miller N, Obrand D. Short-term natural history of isolated gastrocnemius and soleal vein thrombosis. *J. Vasc. Surg.* 2003;37(3):523-7.

[20] Schwarz T, Buschmann L, Beyer J, Halbritter K, Rastan A, Schellong S. Therapy of isolated calf muscle vein thrombosis: a randomized, controlled study. *J. Vasc. Surg.* 2010;52(5):1246-50.

[21] Hirsh J, Lensing AWA. *Vascular Diagnosis.* 1993:779-81.

[22] Bates SM, Jaeschke R, Stevens SM, Goodacre S, Wells PS, Stevenson MD, et al. Diagnosis of dvt: Antithrombotic therapy and prevention of thrombosis, 9th ed: american college of chest physicians evidence-based clinical practice guidelines. *CHEST Journal.* 2012;141(2_suppl):e351S-e418S.

[23] Krünes U, Teubner K, Knipp H, Holzapfel R. Vasa - *Journal of Vascular Diseases.* 1998;27(3):172-5.

[24] Kearon C, Julian JA, Newman TE, Ginsberg JS. *Annals of Internal Medicine.* 1998;128(8):663-77.

[25] Gaitini D. *Journal of Clinical Ultrasound.* 2006;34(6):289-97.

[26] Geerts WH, Bergqvist D, Pineo GF, Heit JA, Samama CM, Lassen MR, et al. Prevention of venous thromboembolism: American College of Chest Physicians Evidence-Based Clinical Practice Guidelines (8th Edition). *Chest.* 2008;133(6 Suppl):381S-453S.

[27] Kearon C, Akl EA, Comerota AJ, Prandoni P, Bounameaux H, Goldhaber SZ, et al. Antithrombotic therapy for vte disease: Antithrombotic therapy and prevention of thrombosis, 9th ed: american college of chest physicians evidence-based clinical practice guidelines. *CHEST Journal.* 2012;141(2_suppl):e419S-e94S.

[28] Dauzat M, Laroche JP, Deklunder G, Ayoub J, Quere I, Lopez FM, et al. Diagnosis of acute lower limb deep venous thrombosis with ultrasound: trends and controversies. *J. Clin. Ultrasound.* 1997;25(7):343-58.

[29] Kearon C, Julian JA, Newman TE, Ginsberg JS. Noninvasive diagnosis of deep venous thrombosis. McMaster Diagnostic Imaging Practice Guidelines Initiative. *Ann. Intern. Med.* 1998;128(8):663-77.

[30] Birdwell BG, Raskob GE, Whitsett TL, Durica SS, Comp PC, George JN, et al. The clinical validity of normal compression ultrasonography in outpatients suspected of having deep venous thrombosis. *Ann. Intern. Med.* 1998;128(1):1-7.

[31] Bernardi E, Camporese G, Buller HR, Siragusa S, Imberti D, Berchio A, et al. Serial 2-point ultrasonography plus D-dimer vs whole-leg color-coded Doppler ultrasonography for diagnosing suspected symptomatic deep vein thrombosis: a randomized controlled trial. *JAMA.* 2008;300(14):1653-9.

[32] Wells PS, Anderson DR, Rodger M, Forgie M, Kearon C, Dreyer J, et al. Evaluation of D-dimer in the diagnosis of suspected deep-vein thrombosis. *N. Engl. J. Med.* 2003;349(13):1227-35.

[33] Wells PS, Anderson DR, Bormanis J, Guy F, Mitchell M, Gray L, et al. Value of assessment of pretest probability of deep-vein thrombosis in clinical management. *Lancet.* 1997;350(9094):1795-8.

[34] Masuda EM, Kistner RL. The case for managing calf vein thrombi with duplex surveillance and selective anticoagulation. *Dis. Mon.* 2010; 56(10):601-13.

[35] Falck-Ytter Y, Francis CW, Johanson NA, Curley C, Dahl OE, Schulman S, et al. Prevention of vte in orthopedic surgery patients: Antithrombotic therapy and prevention of thrombosis, 9th ed: american

college of chest physicians evidence-based clinical practice guidelines. *CHEST Journal*. 2012;141(2_suppl):e278S-e325S.

[36] Kahn SR, Lim W, Dunn AS, Cushman M, Dentali F, Akl EA, et al. Prevention of vte in nonsurgical patients: Antithrombotic therapy and prevention of thrombosis, 9th ed: american college of chest physicians evidence-based clinical practice guidelines. *CHEST Journal.* 2012; 141(2_suppl):e195S-e226S.

[37] Schmidt B, Michler R, Klein M, Faulmann G, Weber C, Schellong S. Ultrasound screening for distal vein thrombosis is not beneficial after major orthopedic surgery. A randomized controlled trial. *Thromb. Haemost*. 2003;90(5):949-54.

[38] Azarbal A, Rowell S, Lewis J, Urankar R, Moseley S, Landry G, et al. Duplex ultrasound screening detects high rates of deep vein thromboses in critically ill trauma patients. *J. Vasc. Surg*. 2011;54(3):743-7; discussion 7-8.

[39] Schulman S, Granqvist S, Juhlin-Dannfelt A, Lockner D. Long-term sequelae of calf vein thrombosis treated with heparin or low-dose streptokinase. *Acta Med. Scand.* 1986;219(4):349-57.

[40] Parisi R, Visonà A, Camporese G, Verlato F, Lessiani G, Antignani PL, et al. Isolated distal deep vein thrombosis: Efficacy and safety of a protocol of treatment. Treatment of Isolated Calf Thrombosis (TICT) study. *International Angiology*. 2009;28(1):68-72.

[41] Hull RD, Raskob GE, Hirsh J, Jay RM, Leclerc JR, Geerts WH, et al. Continuous intravenous heparin compared with intermittent subcutaneous heparin in the initial treatment of proximal-vein thrombosis. *N. Engl. J. Med.* 1986;315(18):1109-14.

[42] Hommes DW, Bura A, Mazzolai L, Buller HR, ten Cate JW. Subcutaneous heparin compared with continuous intravenous heparin administration in the initial treatment of deep vein thrombosis. A meta-analysis. *Ann. Intern. Med.* 1992;116(4):279-84.

[43] Prandoni P, Lensing AW, Buller HR, Carta M, Cogo A, Vigo M, et al. Comparison of subcutaneous low-molecular-weight heparin with intravenous standard heparin in proximal deep-vein thrombosis. *Lancet.* 1992;339(8791):441-5.

[44] Riess H, Koppenhagen K, Tolle A, Kemkes-Matthes B, Grave M, Patek F, et al. Fixed-dose, body weight-independent subcutaneous low molecular weight heparin Certoparin compared with adjusted-dose intravenous unfractionated heparin in patients with proximal deep venous thrombosis. *Thromb. Haemost*. 2003;90(2):252-9.

[45] Harenberg J, Schmidt JA, Koppenhagen K, Tolle A, Huisman MV, Buller HR. Fixed-dose, body weight-independent subcutaneous LMW heparin versus adjusted dose unfractionated intravenous heparin in the initial treatment of proximal vencus thrombosis. EASTERN Investigators. *Thromb. Haemost.* 2000;83(5):652-6.

[46] Hirsh J. Comparison of the relative efficacy and safety of low molecular weight heparin and unfractionated heparin for the treatment of venous thrombosis. *Haemostasis.* 1996;26 Suppl 4:189-98.

[47] Howard AW, Aaron SD. Low molecular weight heparin decreases proximal and distal deep venous thrombosis following total knee arthroplasty. A meta-analysis of randomized trials. *Thromb. Haemost.* 1998;79(5):902-6.

[48] Turpie AG, Bauer KA, Eriksson BI, Lassen MR. Fondaparinux vs enoxaparin for the prevention of venous thromboembolism in major orthopedic surgery: a meta-analysis of 4 randomized double-blind studies. *Arch. Intern. Med.* 2002;162(16):1833-40.

[49] Turpie AG, Bauer KA, Eriksson BI, Lassen MR. Superiority of fondaparinux over enoxaparin in preventing venous thromboembolism in major orthopedic surgery using different efficacy end points. *Chest.* 2004;126(2):501-8.

[50] Agnelli G, Bergqvist D, Cohen AT, Gallus AS, Gent M, investigators P. Randomized clinical trial of postoperative fondaparinux versus perioperative dalteparin for prevention of venous thromboembolism in high-risk abdominal surgery. *Br. J. Surg.* 2005;92(10):1212-20.

[51] Turpie AG, Bauer KA, Caprini JA, Comp PC, Gent M, Muntz JE, et al. Fondaparinux combined with intermittent pneumatic compression vs. intermittent pneumatic compression alone for prevention of venous thromboembolism after abdominal surgery: a randomized, double-blind comparison. *J. Thromb. Haemost.* 2007;5(9):1854-61.

[52] Weitz JI, Eikelboom JW, Samama MM, American College of Chest P. New antithrombotic drugs: Antithrombotic Therapy and Prevention of Thrombosis, 9th ed: American College of Chest Physicians Evidence-Based Clinical Practice Guidelines. *Chest.* 2012;141(2 Suppl):e120S-51S.

[53] van Gogh I, Buller HR, Cohen AT, Davidson B, Decousus H, Gallus AS, et al. Idraparinux versus standard therapy for venous thromboembolic disease. *N. Engl. J. Med.* 2007;357(11):1094-104.

[54] Equinox I. Efficacy and safety of once weekly subcutaneous idrabiotaparinux in the treatment of patients with symptomatic deep venous thrombosis. *J. Thromb. Haemost.* 2011;9(1):92-9.

[55] Paty I, Trellu M, Destors JM, Cortez P, Boelle E, Sanderink G. Reversibility of the anti-FXa activity of idrabiotaparinux (biotinylated idraparinux) by intravenous avidin infusion. *J. Thromb. Haemost.* 2010;8(4):722-9.

[56] Cohen A, Drost P, Marchant N, Mitchell S, Orme M, Rublee D, et al. The efficacy and safety of pharmacological prophylaxis of venous thromboembolism following elective knee or hip replacement: systematic review and network meta-analysis. *Clin. Appl. Thromb. Hemost.* 2012;18(6):611-27.

[57] Gomez-Outes A, Terleira-Fernandez AI, Suarez-Gea ML, Vargas-Castrillon E. Dabigatran, rivaroxaban, or apixaban versus enoxaparin for thromboprophylaxis after total hip or knee replacement: systematic review, meta-analysis, and indirect treatment comparisons. *BMJ.* 2012;344:e3675.

[58] Agnelli G, Gallus A, Goldhaber SZ, Haas S, Huisman MV, Hull RD, et al. Treatment of proximal deep-vein thrombosis with the oral direct factor Xa inhibitor rivaroxaban (BAY 59-7939): the ODIXa-DVT (Oral Direct Factor Xa Inhibitor BAY 59-7939 in Patients With Acute Symptomatic Deep-Vein Thrombosis) study. *Circulation.* 2007; 116(2):180-7.

[59] Duggan ST. Rivaroxaban: a review of its use for the prophylaxis of venous thromboembolism after total hip or knee replacement surgery. *Am. J. Cardiovasc. Drugs*. 2012;12(1):57-72.

[60] Lassen MR, Ageno W, Borris LC, Lieberman JR, Rosencher N, Bandel TJ, et al. Rivaroxaban versus enoxaparin for thromboprophylaxis after total knee arthroplasty. *N. Engl. J. Med.* 2008;358(26):2776-86.

[61] Turpie AG, Lassen MR, Davidson BL, Bauer KA, Gent M, Kwong LM, et al. Rivaroxaban versus enoxaparin for thromboprophylaxis after total knee arthroplasty (RECORD4): a randomised trial. *Lancet.* 2009; 373(9676):1673-80.

[62] Schulman S, Kearon C, Kakkar AK, Mismetti P, Schellong S, Eriksson H, et al. Dabigatran versus warfarin in the treatment of acute venous thromboembolism. *N. Engl. J. Med.* 2009;361(24):2342-52.

[63] McKenna R, Galante J, Bachmann F, Wallace DL, Kaushal PS, Meredith P. Prevention of venous thromboembolism after total knee

replacement by high-dose aspirin or intermittent calf and thigh compression. *Br. Med. J.* 1980;280(6213):514-7.

[64] Collaborative overview of randomised trials of antiplatelet therapy--III: Reduction in venous thrombosis and pulmonary embolism by antiplatelet prophylaxis among surgical and medical patients. Antiplatelet Trialists' Collaboration. *BMJ*. 1994;308(6923):235-46.

[65] Prevention of pulmonary embolism and deep vein thrombosis with low dose aspirin: Pulmonary Embolism Prevention (PEP) trial. *Lancet*. 2000;355(9212):1295-302.

[66] Powers PJ, Gent M, Jay RM, Julian DH, Turpie AG, Levine M, et al. A randomized trial of less intense postoperative warfarin or aspirin therapy in the prevention of venous thromboembolism after surgery for fractured hip. *Arch. Intern. Med.* 1989;149(4):771-4.

[67] Gent M, Hirsh J, Ginsberg JS, Powers PJ, Levine MN, Geerts WH, et al. Low-molecular-weight heparinoid orgaran is more effective than aspirin in the prevention of venous thromboembolism after surgery for hip fracture. *Circulation*. 1996;93(1):80-4.

[68] Ogawa T, Hoshino S, Midorikawa H, Sato K. Intermittent pneumatic compression of the foot and calf improves the outcome of catheter-directed thrombolysis using low-dose urokinase in patients with acute proximal venous thrombosis of the leg. *J. Vasc. Surg*. 2005;42(5):940-4.

[69] Elliott CG, Dudney TM, Egger M, Orme JF, Clemmer TP, Horn SD, et al. Calf-thigh sequential pneumatic compression compared with plantar venous pneumatic compression to prevent deep-vein thrombosis after non-lower extremity trauma. *J. Trauma*. 1999;47(1):25-32.

[70] Warwick D, Harrison J, Glew D, Mitchelmore A, Peters TJ, Donovan J. Comparison of the use of a foot pump with the use of low-molecular-weight heparin for the prevention of deep-vein thrombosis after total hip replacement. A prospective, randomized trial. *J. Bone Joint Surg. Am.* 1998;80(8):1158-66.

[71] Urbankova J, Quiroz R, Kucher N, Goldhaber SZ. Intermittent pneumatic compression and deep vein thrombosis prevention. A meta-analysis in postoperative patients. *Thromb. Haemost*. 2005;94(6):1181-5.

[72] Roderick P, Ferris G, Wilson K, Halls H, Jackson D, Collins R, et al. Towards evidence-based guidelines for the prevention of venous thromboembolism: systematic reviews of mechanical methods, oral anticoagulation, dextran and regional anaesthesia as thromboprophylaxis. *Health Technol. Assess*. 2005;9(49):iii-iv, ix-x, 1-78.

[73] Collaboration CT. Thigh-length versus below-knee stockings for deep venous thrombosis prophylaxis after stroke: a randomized trial. *Ann. Intern. Med.* 2010;153(9):553-62.

In: Venous Thrombosis
Editor: Caroline H. Gutmann

ISBN: 978-1-63117-293-9

Chapter 3

Deep Venous Thrombosis as a Complication of Surgery and Trauma

Khanjan H. Nagarsheth, M.D. and Kuldeep Singh, M.D.
Staten Island University Hospital,
Division of Vascular Surgery, Staten Island, NY, US

Abstract

The incidence of deep venous thrombosis (DVT) in the surgical population varies by type of patient and surgical procedure, contributing an unknown percentile of the overall estimated 250,000 DVTs annually.

Most DVTs are proximal and are found above the knee in the iliac, femoral, or popliteal veins. Those found below the knee, in any of the three groups of paired deep calf veins, are typically considered of less clinical significance. Upper extremity DVTs, in the axillary and subclavian veins, account for 5% of DVTs and are seen most often in the surgical patient associated with indwelling catheters or in patients with malignancy; 30% of these DVTs are estimated to lead to pulmonary embolism (PE). Risk factors for DVT include advanced age, malignancy, immobilization, trauma, oral contraceptives, hormone replacement, pregnancy, obesity, neurologic or cardiac disease, prolonged travel, and inflammatory states. A recent review of 1,485 spinal surgery patients found similar factors such as active malignancy, prior DVT or PE, estrogen replacement therapy, and renal disease to be significant on univariate analysis.

Interestingly, on multivariate analysis, estrogen replacement therapy and discharge to a rehabilitation facility had the strongest correlations as risk factors for DVT or PE.

A high index of suspicion is necessary for early diagnosis of this condition. Signs and symptoms include pain, edema usually of the calf or ankle, and warmth or erythema of the skin over the thrombosis. More than 50% of DVTs are asymptomatic and found solely on imaging. Duplex ultrasound imaging is highly sensitive and specific. Laboratory tests such as D-dimer can be useful adjuncts in making the diagnosis of DVT, although this is not as sensitive or specific for the disease as duplex ultrasonography.

The goal of DVT treatment is to reduce the risk of PE, decrease extension of DVT, and prevent the almost 30% recurrence rate of an untreated DVT. Systemic anticoagulation is the mainstay of treatment in patients diagnosed with DVT and PE. Catheter directed pharmacologic thrombolysis is another option that is thought to preserve valve function. Inferior vena cava (IVC) filter placement is another aspect of DVT treatment.

Introduction

Deep venous thrombosis (DVT) is a well-described entity that affects the extremity deep venous system. Overall DVT is noted affect approximately 56 per 100,000 people per year. The incidence of DVT in the surgical population varies by type of patient and surgical procedure, contributing an unknown percentile of the overall estimated 250,000 DVTs annually. A meta-analysis found that high-risk general surgery patients have a 20% risk of a proximal DVT [1]. Hull et al. found the overall incidence of DVT to be 19% in the general surgical patient, 24% in patients undergoing elective neurosurgical procedures, between 48% and 61% in those undergoing lower extremity orthopedic procedures [2]. Most deep venous thromboses that occur in the surgical patient are believed to develop in the operating room and the remainder occurs during the first few days post-operative. One population-based study determined that hospitalized patients had more than a 100-fold increase in the incidence of venous thromboembolism compared to the general populous [3].

Most DVTs are proximal, found above the knee in the iliac, femoral, or popliteal veins.

Deep venous thrombosis below the knee can occur in any of the three groups of paired deep calf veins however the significance of this subgroup is still unclear.

Upper extremity DVTs, in the axillary and subclavian veins, account for 5% of DVTs and are seen most often in the surgical patient associated with indwelling catheters or in patients with malignancy. Up to 10% of upper extremity deep venous thromboses are believed to lead to pulmonary embolism (PE). [4]

Phlegmasia alba dolens describes the condition of an extremely swollen and painful leg with pitting edema, that blanches as a result of iliofemoral venous system obstruction. If this continues to compromise arterial inflow, phegmasia cerulea dolens, a painful blue leg, can develop, and this can be a surgical emergency.

Risk Factors

Rudolf Virchow's first proposed his theory for the cause of venous thrombosis in 1856. This so-called triad involved venous stasis, changes in the endothelial lining of the vein and underlying hypercoaguability, and still relevant in discussing the etiology of DVTs in surgical and trauma patients [5]. The first component of the triad is venous stasis. Venous stasis is believed to begin at the vein valves. Venography has revealed that contrast medium remains stagnant at the venous valvular sinuses and takes an average of 27 minutes to clear [6]. This valvular sinus stasis is associated with hypoxia and a local increase in hematocrit that creates a hypercoaguable setting and promotes thrombosis.

Another aspect that contributes to venous stasis is a loss of the calf-muscle pump often seen in non-ambulatory, immobilized critically ill patients. The calf veins normally fill with between 100 mL and 150 mL of blood and muscle contraction results in the feeding perforator vein valves being forced closed. This causes the blood to be forced proximally through outflow valves towards the heart, against gravity.

The second part of the triad is changes in the vein's endothelial lining, most commonly in the form of endothelial injury. Research has shown that injury to veins, such as microscopic tears within valve cusps, occur at sites distal to the surgery. This endothelial layer normally serves a vasodilatory function and provides a localized fibrinolytic milieu that prevents thrombus formation.

Under normal conditions, the endothelium produces thrombomodulin, heparin sulfate, dermatan sulfate, tissue plasminogen activator and a number of other cytokines and molecules that prevent platelet activation and adhesion. When this endothelial layer is disturbed, an inflammatory cascade ensues and results in vasoconstriction and exposure of tissue factor with upregulation of von Willebrand factor, activated Factor V and tissue factor. These events contribute to venous thrombosis.

Lastly, there is a known hypercoaguable state that occurs after surgery. Injured cells release the procoagulant tissue factor. Physiologic stresses, like surgery or trauma, also are associated with increased platelet count, adhesiveness, changes in the coagulation cascade, and endogenous fibrinolytic activity. All three of these factors are actually present in many post-surgical patients.

There are a number of acquired prothrombotic risk factors that include: advanced age, malignancy, immobilization, oral contraceptives, hormone replacement, pregnancy, obesity, neurologic or cardiac disease, prolonged travel, and inflammatory states.

Hypercoaguable conditions can simultaneously be present in critically ill and post-operative patients. These include: antithrombin deficiency, protein C and S deficiency, factor V Leiden, prothrombin 20210A gene mutation, blood group non-O, dysfibrinogenemia, dysplasminogenemia, hyperhomocystinemia, reduced heparin cofactor II activity, elevated levels of clotting factors, and elevated plasminogen activator inhibitor [7].

A recent review of 1,485 spinal surgery patients found similar factors such as active maligancy, prior DVT or PE, estrogen replacement therapy, and renal disease to be significant on univariate analysis. Interestingly, on multivariate analysis, estrogen replacement therapy and discharge to a rehabilitation facility had the strongest correlations as risk factors for DVT or PE. [8]

Diagnosis

Physical exam often causes the provider to investigate for presence of a DVT. A high index of suspicion is needed for prompt diagnosis and subsequent treatment of this condition. Signs and symptoms such as pain, edema of the calf or ankle, and warmth or erythema of the skin should alert the healthcare team to possible presence of DVT. However, more than 50% of DVTs are asymptomatic and found solely on imaging.

Venous duplex ultrasound imaging has a very high sensitivity and is greater than 95% specific for DVT [9].

Some of its advantages to other diagnostic modalities include: no need for intravenous contrast, being relatively painless, safe pregnant patients and non-invasive. Duplex ultrasonography assesses for the presence of thrombus, venous dilation, and venous segment incompressibility. The chronicity of DVT can be assessed by the absence of spontaneous flow, loss flow variation with respiration, failure to increase flow with distal augmentation, and characterization of the thrombus as having increased echogenicity and heterogenicity. Venous duplex ultrasound is not ideal in identifying thrombus in the pelvic and central venous systems. Therefore, when assessing for pelvic vein, superior and inferior vena cava thrombus, magnetic resonance venography or CT venogram may be useful in securing the diagnosis.

Deep venous thrombosis is identified by autopsy in over 60% of trauma victims. A recent large retrospective review sought to determine the value of routine ultrasound surveillence to identify DVTs and found that it is warranted in the highest risk patients. Moderate risk patients had no benefit from routine surveillance ultrasound over those performed based on clinical suspicion [10].

Laboratory tests such as D-dimer can be useful adjuncts in making the diagnosis of DVT, but lack the sensitivity or specificity that is afforded by duplex ultrasonography. D-dimer assay test measures cross-linked fibrin degradation products. This is used in place of plasmin's activity on fibrin. D-dimer is often elevated stressed states. Therefore, only a negative result has any clinical significance in the evaluation of DVT in a surgical patient or trauma victim.

Prophylaxis

Prophylaxis in the peri-operative patient has been shown to be effective in reducing the rates of DVTs and pulmonary embolisms (PE). Prophylaxis can be either pharmacologic or mechanical in nature. Typically, pharmacologic options include low molecular weight heparin that inhibits factor Xa and IIa, and low dose unfractionated heparin. These pharmacological forms of prophylaxis have been shown to reduce the incidence of post-operative DVTs from 25% to 8% [1]. Mechanical prophylaxis includes intermittent pneumatic compression or sequential compression devices. These methods help to decrease venous stasis and help to increase fibrinolysis, by their actions on plasminogen activator inhibitor-1.

Early ambulation can also help in DVT prevention. Patients who are undergoing major abdominal or orthopedic surgery, those who have sustained major trauma, or will be immobile for more than three days are all suitable for mechanical prophylaxis.

Treatment

The therapeutic goal of DVT treatment is to reduce the risk of PE, decrease extension of DVT, and prevent the recurrence of DVTs. The recurrence rate of untreated DVT has been quoted as high as 30% in the literature.

Systemic anticoagulation is the mainstay of treatment in patients with DVT and PE who do not have a contra-indication. Unfractionated heparin (UFH) administered as a continuous intravenous drip followed by warfarin administration, is the most common regimen for treatment. Warfarin must be started only after heparin is initiated, to avoid the risk of warfarin-induced skin necrosis. This phenomenon is caused by the transient hypercoaguable state that is induced by protein C and S levels diminishing before other vitamin K dependent factors. Monitoring of the partial thromboplastin time is important for patients receiving an intravenous infusion of heparin.

Low molecular weight heparin (LMWH) has been shown to have a lower bleeding risk than UFH and be equal or superior in preventing recurrence of DVT compared to UFH. Low molecular weight heparin also has a decreased mortality rate, and lower incidence of heparin induced thrombocytopenia and thrombosis (HITT) than UFH. There is less interference with protein C and more predictable bioavailability associated with LMWH. The mechanism of action includes greater anti-factor Xa and less direct anti-thrombin inhibition. Monitoring for LMWH was not routinely done, but some situations now need intermittent measurement of anti-factor Xa levels. These situations include pediatric, pregnant, obese and renal failure patients.

There is also a class of drugs called direct factor Xa inhibitors have received significant attention, including: rivaroxaban [11], fondaparinux, and dabigatran. These agents do not use antithrombin as a mediator. The duration of systemic anticoagulation is typically three months for an initial proximal DVT. Lifelong therapy is recommended after a second DVT or PE and for those associated with non-temporary hypercoaguable states such as malignancy or genetic diagnoses. Treatment for more distal DVTs in calf veins should also be for three months [12].

Catheter directed pharmacologic thrombolysis is uncommonly used but when initiated early, usually within two week of symptoms, is thought to preserve valve function.

This is performed generally with recombinant tissue plasminogen activator (tPA). Indications include high volume iliofemoral DVT, phlegmasia, and thrombosis with ischemia or vascular compromise.

Axillary or subclavian DVTs in young patients with effort thrombosis, or Paget-Schrotter syndrome, may improve venous patency and decrease post-thrombotic syndrome. Endovascular and surgical methods are also used and can include thrombectomy, angioplasty, and stenting.

Patients with DVTs should also be encouraged to wear compression stockings, elevate the extremity at rest, and ambulate frequently.

Inferior vena cava (IVC) filter placement is another possible DVT treatment. They can be placed before a DVT is diagnosed, or after, to prevent PE. The indications for IVC filter placement are recurrent venous thrombo-embolism while on adequate anticoagulation, a new DVT with a contra-indication to anticoagulation, complications of anticoagulation treatment, or extension of iliofemoral DVT during anticoagulation.

There is an approximate 4% recurrence rate, and a 95% patency rate. Retrievable IVC filters can be utilized in multiple trauma victims and in high-risk surgical patients.

A number of recent studies have shown excellent retrieval rates for retrievable filters, when a registry is initiated and maintained to keep track of these patients [13].

Complications of DVT

The natural history of DVTs can take one of several routes. They can lend way to thromboembolization in the form of a PE, which can be highly morbid and potentially fatal.

Next DVTs can result in luminal recanalization or can lead to chronic occlusion with scarring. Partial lumen patency can be restored but intraluminal scarring can trap valves, causing valvular incompetence. Valve incompetence and vein wall fibrosis can manifest, early on, as edema, pain, and immobility.

Eventually chronic venous insufficiency with valvular dysfunction develops and is defined as post thrombotic syndrome. There is an overall estimated 9% fatality rate after first time DVT [1].

Complications of Treatment

There have been a number of studies that have looked into the risk of venous thromboembolism in trauma patients, but there are relatively few that have examined bleeding complications associated with thromboprophylaxis in this patient population.

One prospective study looked at patients with traumatic brain injury and risk of major bleeding associated with thromboprophylaxis within 48 hours of admission. In this review 3.4% of patients were noted to have progression of hemorrhage found on CT scan and 1.1% of patients had a change in management or outcome based on this bleeding. [14]

In the patient undergoing general abdominal and pelvic surgery, there is a paucity of data on the risk factors for bleeding complications associated with thromboprophylaxis. Based on data collected by the American College of Chest Physicians for their 2012 supplement on prevention of venous thromboembolism in surgical patients, they found a major bleeding risk 0.7 to 1.2% in this population, associated with thrombophrophylaxis. They also estimated a major bleeding risk of 1.8 times greater in high risk patients when compared to control groups. [15]

Treatment and prophylaxis for DVT is also associated with certain complications. There is up to a 9% risk of bleeding in the first five days of UFH administration when therapeutic PTT levels are achieved. Heparin Induced Thrombotic Thrombocytopenia occurs 0.6-30% per year. and is caused by heparin-dependent antibody IgG which binds to platelets causing aggregation. Signs and symptoms typically start 3-14 days after starting heparin and include: >50% drop in platelets from baseline, or evidence of new thrombosis while on heparin therapy. Diagnosis is confirmed by ELISA for antiheparin antibody. Heparin should be stopped if HITT is suspected and a direct thrombin inhibitor like lepirudin or argatroban or a Factor Xa inhibitor such as fondaparinux or rivaroxaban is initiated for anticoagulation.

Conclusion

Deep venous thrombosis is a significant problem affecting post-operative patients and those who sustain serious trauma. Early detection and diagnosis are important so therapy can be initiated to prevent further complications such as extension or thromboembolism.

Therapy can be either pharmacologic or mechanical, and some patients may require further surgical intervention if they have a large clot burden.

References

[1] Geerts, W. H., Heit, J. A., Clagett, G. P., et al. Prevention of venous thromboembolism. *Chest* 2001;119:132S.

[2] Hull, R. D., Raskob, G. E., Hirsh, J. Prophylaxis of venous thromboembolism. An overview. *Chest*. 1986;89 (5 Suppl.):374S-383S.

[3] Heit, J. A., Melton, L. J. 3rd, Lohse, C. M., et al. Incidence of venous thromboembolism in hospitalized patients vs community residents. *Mayo Clin. Proc*. 2001;76(1):1102-10.

[4] Lee, J. A., Zierler, B. K., Zierler, R. E. The risk factors and clinical outcomes of upper extremity deep venous thrombosis. *Vasc. Endovascular Surg*. 2012 Feb.;46(2):139-44.

[5] Esmon, C. T. Basic mechanism and pathogenesis of venous thrombosis. *Blood Rev*. 2009;23(5): 225-9.

[6] McLachlin, A. D., McLachlin, J. A., Jory, T. A., Rawling, E. G. Venous stasis in the lower extremities. *Ann. Surg*. 1960;152:678-83.

[7] Goldhaber, S. Z., Bounameaux, H. Pulmonary embolism and deep vein thrombosis. *Lancet*. 2012;12(9828):1835-46.

[8] Schulte, L. M., O'Brien, J. R., Beans, M. C., et al. Deep venous thrombosis and pulmonary embolism after spine surgery: Incidence and patient risk factors. *Am. J. Orthop*. 2013;42(6):267-270.

[9] Douglas, M. G., Sumner, D. S. Duplex scanning for deep vein thrombosis: has it replaced both phlebography and noninvasive testing? *Semin. Vasc. Surg*. 1996;9:3.

[10] Bandle, J., Shackford, S. R., Kahl, J. E., Sise, C. B., Calvo, R. Y., Shackford, M. C., Sise, M. J. The value of lower-extremity duplex surveillance to detect deep vein thrombosis in trauma patients. *J. Trauma Acute Care Surg*. 2013;74(2):575-80.

[11] EINSTEIN Investigators, Bauersachs, R., Berkowitz, S. D., Brenner, B., Buller, H. R., et al. Oral Rivaroxaban for Symptomatic Venous Thromboembolism. *N. Engl. J. Med.* 2010;363:2499-2510.

[12] Hirsch, J., Guyatt, G., Albers, G. W., Harrington, R., Schunemann, H. J. Antithrombotic and thrombolytic therapy American College of Chest Physicians evidence based clinical practice guidelines (8th edition). *Chest* 2008; 133:110S–112S.

[13] Lucas, D. J., Dunne, J. R., Rodriguez, C. J., et al. Dedicated tracking of patients with retrievable inferior vena cava filters improved retrieval rates. *Am. Surg*. 2012;78(8):870-4.

[14] Norwood, S. H., Berne, J. D., Rowe, S. A., Villarreal, D. H., Ledlie, J. T. Early venous thromboembolism prophylaxis with enoxaparin in patients with blunt traumatic brain injury. *J. Trauma* 2008;65(5):1021-1026.

[15] Gould, M. K., Garcia, D. A., Wren, S. M., et al. Prevention of VTE in nonorthopedic surgical patients: Antithrombotic therapy and prevention of thrombosis, 9th ed: American College of Chest Physicians evidence-based clinical practice guidelines. *Chest* 2012;114 (2 Suppl.):e227S-77S.

In: Venous Thrombosis
Editor: Caroline H. Gutmann
ISBN: 978-1-63117-293-9

Chapter 4

Superficial Thrombophlebitis

Khanjan H. Nagarsheth, M.D. and Kuldeep Singh, M.D.
Staten Island University Hospital,
Division of Vascular Surgery, Staten Island, NY, US

Abstract

Superficial thrombophlebitis is defined as inflammation and thrombosis of a vein near the skin's surface. Most studies underestimate the occurrence of superficial thormbophlebitis and although the greater or lesser saphenous veins are the most commonly affected veins, this disease can occur at any part of the body.

This condition is often associated with a long term intravenous (IV) catheter and is differentiated from septic thrombophlebitis by the absence of systemic signs of infection. Risk factors include recent venous catheterization, a history of previous superficial venous thrombosis, DVT or PE, recent surgery, trauma, pregnancy, high dose estrogen therapy, immobilization, malignancy, varicose veins, obesity, or intravenous drug abuse.

Superficial thrombophlebitis remains a clinical diagnosis. Symptoms include localized pain and warmth over the site and patients will present with tenderness to palpation, induration, and erythema over a palpable cord. It is noted that superficial thrombophlebitis coexists with DVT in up to 53% of cases and PE in up to 33% of cases. Superficial thrombophlebitis can progress rapidly to venous thromboembolism (VTE) in as much as 15% of cases.

Even though most times superficial thrombophlebitis will resolve on its own, it is not considered to be self limited and complications can occur. These include extension from a superficial vein to a deep vein, postphlebitic syndrome, chronic DVTs, suppurative thrombophlebilitis and septic thrombophlebitis.

The aim of treatment is to alleviate symptoms and prevent extension to deep veins. The mainstay of treatment consists of extremity elevation, warm compresses, and the use of non-steroidal anti-inflammatory drugs (NSAID). Most patients respond to this conservative management regime with symptom resolution or improvement in 7-10 days. There is some evidence that shows the use of subtherapeutic doses of low molecular weight heparin can help in prevention of extension of superficial thrombophlebitis to DVT but there are no large multicenter trials to support this and make it standard of care.

Introduction

Superficial thrombophlebitis (ST), otherwise known as superficial venous thrombosis or superficial phlebitis is an inflammatory-thrombosis process of a vein near the skin's surface. These patients present with localized pain, erythema, warmth and tenderness along the course of the vein. ST is believed to occur with an incidence of 125,000 cases per year [1]. The incidence of ST increases with age. Superficial thrombophlebitis is described to increase in incidence in males from 0.05 per 1000 per year in the third decade of life to 1.8 per 1000 per year in the eighth decade of life [2]. The actual morbidity associated with ST is under-represented in the literature, as most studies have excluded patients with concomitantly occurring, past history of, or family history of venous thromboembolism (VTE).

The greater saphenous (GSV) and superficial saphenous veins (SSV) are the most commonly affected veins with ST. One study found that the GSV was affected in 63.4% of patients, whereas the SSV was affected in 14.2% of cases. [3] Superficial thrombophlebitis can also occur in veins of the abdomen, thorax, genitals or neck. Mondor's disease is ST of the superficial veins of the breast or penis. The upper, outer quadrant of the breast is most commonly affected by ST, but it can also occur along the submammary fold and costal margin. When this is clinically encountered, malignancy should be suspected. Penile Mondor's disease, usually of the dorsal vein, is caused by trauma or repetition injury.

Septic thrombophlebitis is differentiated from ST by having signs of an infection.

Patients will frequently present with systemic symptoms of fevers, rigors and chills. There is often presence of an antecedent long-term intravenous catheter such as a peripherally inserted central catheter (PICC). Suppurative thrombophlebitis occurs when there is purulence within a vein. This condition can lead to septicemia and even death.

Risk Factors

Superficial thrombophlebitis occurs as a result of three major risk factors. The first risk factor is often seen in surgical patients. This condition is often associated with indwelling catheters, such as PICC lines and intravenous catheters. These lines result in endothelial damage, which predisposes the patient to thrombosis. The next risk factor is seen as a result of an underlying hypercoaguable disorder or autoimmune diseases, such as anti-phospholipid syndrome or systemic lupus erythematosus. The third risk factor is associated with venous stasis and is often seen in patients with venous varicosities.

Patients frequently have a history of previous superficial venous thrombosis, VTE, recent surgery or trauma, pregnancy, oral contraceptive medications, immobilization, malignancy, obesity, or intravenous drug abuse [4]. The inciting event (trauma, catheterization, etc.) triggers an inflammatory cascade involving platelet adhesion. Thromboxane A2 and thrombin are involved in this inflammatory cascade and increase platelet aggregation.

Diagnosis

Superficial thrombophlebitis is a clinical diagnosis and the symptoms include localized pain and warmth over the site. Often patients have tenderness to palpation, induration, and erythema over a palpable cord. Edema is found in patients that have an underlying deep venous thrombosis. Superficial thrombophlebitis can have a delayed presentation, after the intravenous catheter has been removed, and can take many months to completely resolve. Since these findings can be somewhat non-specific, a thorough differential diagnosis should be investigated. This differential includes: ascending lymphangitis, cellulitis, erythema nodosum, and panniculitis. A venous duplex ultrasound (VDUS) can show thickened and non-compressible superficial veins. Dilated veins and hypoechoic lumens identify Acute ST on VDUS.

Duplex ultrasound can accurately show the extent of involvement of the superficial and deep venous systems and as such should be used to also rule out a DVT. Since VDUS is relatively inexpensive and noninvasive, it can be repeated to follow the progression or resolution of ST.

In the literature, ST coexists with DVT in as much as 53% of cases and PE in almost one-third of cases. Superficial thrombophlebitis can progress rapidly to venous thromboembolism (VTE) in as many as 15% of cases [5]. Given these high rates of dual diagnosis, VTE should be worked up when ST is identified. Some have advocated assuming concurrent VTE and treating with anticoagulation, especially in those with high clinical risk factors. Superficial thrombophlebitis is also associated with various vasculitides, such as Buerger's disease and polyarteritis nodosa, which may be concurrently present.

Complications

Superficial thrombophlebitis often resolves spontaneously, but when it is not self-limiting, various complications can develop. Extension to the deep venous system results in DVT formation.

When the vein recanalizes leading to a valveless channel, that vein is now susceptible to a postphlebitic syndrome similar to postthrombotic syndrome after chronic DVTs. Postphlebitic syndrome manifests with pain, edema, hyperpigmentation, ulceration, and an increased risk of recurrence. Superficial thrombophlebitis can convert to septic or suppurative thrombophlebitis; which can lead to septicemia, septic emboli, and metastatic abscess formation. The most common organisms isolated from suppurative thrombophlebitis include Staphylooccus aureus, Pseudomonas spp, Escherichia coli and Klebsiella spp [6].

Treatment

The aim of treatment is to alleviate symptoms and prevent extension to deep veins. The specific treatment of ST should be tailored based on the etiology and location of the thrombosis. The mainstay of treatment consists of extremity elevation, warm compresses, and the use of non-steroidal anti-inflammatory drugs (NSAID).

Adjunct elements such as compression stockings or wraps and regular ambulation have also been shown to be helpful. There are also reports of topical anticoagulants (heparin gel) can decrease complications. Most patients respond to this conservative management regime with symptom resolution or improvement in 7-10 days. Venous duplex can be performed to confirm resolution or progression of disease. As mentioned earlier, hypercoaguable states can precede ST and so a hypercoaguable work up is indicated in some patients. Patients who should definitely undergo this work up include those with recurrent ST, extensive affected segments, unusual locations, and spontaneous thromboses without obvious risk factors.

Suppurative and septic thrombophlebitis requires a more aggressive course of action, as they are associated with more dire consequences. Antibiotic therapy targeted to the presumed underlying organism should be initiated promptly. Selective excision of the vein along its course may also be necessary to remove the nidus of infection, prevent bacteremia and subsequent septicemia.

Excision may also be indicated for recurrent superficial thrombophlebitis along the same vein segment. However in these cases, it is best if surgery can wait until the inflammation is resolved.

Some advocate treating all ST as VTE, and start anticoagulation promptly. If a patient is considered high risk for anticoagulation or very low risk for VTE, an ultrasound can be repeated in five to seven days to evaluate for progression of disease before starting anticoagulation. The STENOX (Superficial thrombophlebitis Treated by Enoxaparin) study compared placebo to treatment with subtherapuetic enoxaparin for less than 2 weeks. The patients who received treatment decreased extension and relapse rates in the short term, but this benefit of treatment with enoxaparin was lost by the six month follow up visit [7].

Similarly, Decousus et al. looked at using fondaparinux (2.5mg) for 45 days of treatment. These treated patients experienced a significant decrease in progression of thrombosis, recurrence, and new VTE over placebo during the study period and for 30 days of follow up after [8]. Recurrence is reported as 15-20%. One study found that 10% of subjects still developed VTE within three months despite anticoagulation, with an increase seen in patients with prior VTE, malignancy, or male gender [9].

For patients suffering from a symptomatic thrombosed saphenous vein surgical options utilized in the past included: saphenofemoral surgical disconnection, ligation of the greater saphenous vein (GSV), surgical removal of thrombus in the GSV, or excision of the GSV.

Surgery acts to provoke further thrombosis, increases health care costs, and has an increased rate of complications. Therefore surgery has largely been abandoned in the treatment of ST [10].

Conclusion

Patients with ST should be stratified based on risk factors for developing complications. This risk stratification and identification of risk factors should help guide treatment options.

These treatment options can vary from surveillance and conservative measures to full anticoagulation and possible surgery depending on location of the pathology and degree of symptoms.

References

[1] Vitt, M. J., Barnes, R. W. Nonoperative treatment of acute superficial thrombophlebitis and deep femoral venous thrombosis. In: Ernst, C. B. Stanley, J. C., eds. *Current therapy in vascular surgery*. St. Louis: Mosby; 1995, p. 888.

[2] Coon, W. W., Willis, P. W., Keller, J. B. Venous thromboembolism and other venous disease in the Tecumseh community health study. *Circulation* 1973;48:839-846.

[3] Quere, I., Leizorcovicz, A., Galanaud, J. P., et al. Superficial venous thrombosis and compression ultrasound imaging. *J. Vasc. Surg*. 2012;56 (4):1032-8.e1.

[4] Lutter, K. S., Kerr, T. M., Roedersheimer, L. R., Lohr, J. M., Sampson, M. G. Superficial Thrombophlebitis diagnosed by duplex scanning. *Surgery* 1991;110(1):42–6.

[5] Leon, L., Giannoukas, A. D., Dodd, D., Chan, P., Labropoulos, N. Clinical significance of superficial vein thrombosis. *Eur. J. Vasc. Endovasc. Surg*. 2005;29(1):10-17.

[6] Brook, I., Frazier, E. H. Aerobic and anaerobic microbiology of superficial suppurative thrombophlebitis. *Arch. Surg*. 1996;131(1):95-7.

[7] Superficial thrombophlebitis Treated by Enoxaparin study group: A pilot randomized double-blind comparison ofa ow molecular-weight heparin, a nonsteroidal antiinflammatory agent, and placebo in treatment of superficial vein thrombosis. *Arch. Intern. Med.* 2003;163:1657-1663.

[8] Decousus, H., Prandoni, P., Mismetti, M., et al. Fondaparinux for the treatment of superficial vein thrombosis in the legs. *N Engl. J. Med.* 2010;363(13):1222-1232.

[9] Decousus, H., Ouere Praslar, E., et al. Superficial venous thrombosis and venous thromboemboism: a large prospective epidemiologic study. *Ann. Intern. Med.* 2010;152(4):218-224.

[10] Lozano, F. S., Almazan, A. Low-molecular-weight heparin versus saphenofemoral disconnection for the treatment of above-knee greater saphenous thrombophlebitis: a prospective study. *Vasc. Endovasc. Surg.* 2003;37(6):415-420.

In: Venous Thrombosis
Editor: Caroline H. Gutmann

ISBN: 978-1-63117-293-9

Chapter 5

Current Knowledge of Genetic Risk Factors for Venous Thrombosis

S. Navarro[1,*], L. Martos[1], E. Bonet[1,2], L. Ramón[1], F. España[1] and P. Medina[1]

[1] Hemostasis, Thrombosis, Arteriosclerosis and Vascular Biology Group, Valencia, Spain

[2] Clinical Pathology Service, La Fe University and Polytechnic Hospital, Valencia, Spain

Abstract

Thrombophilias can be defined as a group of inherited or acquired disorders that increase the risk of developing thrombosis. Venous thromboembolism (VT) is considered a multifactorial disease produced by a sum of risk factors that predispose to the thrombotic event. This predisposition includes genetic and acquired defects. VT is one of the major public health problems worldwide, contributing to an estimated >500,000 deaths in Europe each year, with a mortality rate of 10% [1]. The risk of recurrence is about 6% per year, and post-thrombotic disease

* Corresponding author: Dra. Silvia Navarro, IIS La Fe, Hospital Universitario y Politécnico La Fe, Torre A, 5ª planta, Laboratorio 5.16, Av. Bulevar Sur s/n, 46026 Valencia, Spain. Phone: +34-961246640, Fax: +34-961246620, E-mail: navarro_silros@gva.es.

occurs within the next 5 years following a VT event in about 25% of patients [2, 3]. VT is a common multifactorial disease, with both established environmental and genetic risk factors [4].

The genetic basis of the VT is only partially known, and thrombophilia can only explain around 50% of the thrombotic events. Hence, the known risk factors, together with yet unknown alterations in any component of the haemostatic system, may allow us to further clarify the underlying mechanism of VT. The known genetic risk factors confer a poor relative VT risk, altogether can only explain about 5% of the VT heritability [5].

The identification of disease-associated VT genes suspected to be involved in the physiopathology of the disease could help to define its genetic determinants.

Moreover, the recent availability of high-throughput genotyping technologies and their application in the framework of genome-wide association studies (GWAS) have enabled the identification of novel susceptibility loci [6-12]. From 1965 to 2013, 16 genes/loci have been robustly associated with the susceptibility to VT [5], most of them affecting the coagulation cascade. In addition to the well-known established susceptibility genes for VT: *F5*, *F2*, *FGG*, *PROC*, *PROS*, *SERPINC1*, and ABO blood group, new emerging susceptibility loci have arisen: *C4BPA/C4BPB*, *F11*, *G6P*, *HIVEP1*, *KNG1*, *STXBP5*, *TCN2*, *VWF*. However, independent case-control studies are needed to confirm the association with the disease for these emerging genes. This chapter summarizes the current information on the role of genetic risk factors for venous thrombosis.

1. Well-Established Genetic Risk Factors for Venous Thrombosis

1.1. Factor V Gene

Dahlbäck et al. [13] described three families in whom activated protein C (APC) did not yield the expected prolongation of the clotting time in an activated partial thromboplastin time (aPTT) assay, and defined a new phenotype, called APC resistance (APCR). APCR co-segregates with the Factor V gene (*F5*), in particular with the FV Leiden mutation (g.1691G>T; rs6025), which encodes the substitution of arginine for glutamine at 506 position (R506Q), affecting one of the APC cleavage sites in the FV molecule [14]. This abnormal FV molecule is partially resistant to inactivation by APC, leading to a hypercoagulable state, and is the most common genetic risk factor for familial venous thrombosis [14-16]. In Caucasians, the frequency of the FV Leiden mutation is around 5%, while in patients with VT is 21.0% [17, 18]. The risk of VT in heterozygous carriers of the FV Leiden mutation is approximately five fold higher than in the general population [19].

More recently, Smith et al. [20] identified the *F5* rs4524 variant, a non-synonymous substitution of lysine for arginine at the 858 residue (K858R), as a new VT-associated SNP. This SNP in *F5* was consistently associated with VT in three large Dutch case–control studies (MEGA-$_2$ OR=1.21; 95% CI=1.10-1.34; P<0.001), and linkage disequilibrium between this mutation and the FV Leiden was low ($r2$ = 0.02) [21]. In two French GWAS analyses, the OR for VT associated with the rs4524 allele was 1.17 (P = 0.013; PE Morange, DA Tregouet, unpublished data). The functionality of the rs4524 remains to be addressed.

When FV Leiden mutation is present in combination with other genetic risk factors, such as the presence of prothrombin 20210A mutation, haplotypes of the EPCR gene (*PROCR*) [22], or the ABO blood group [23], the risk of VT is modified, thus confirming the multifactorial origin of thrombosis.

1.2. Prothrombin Gene

Prothrombin (FII) has procoagulant, anticoagulant, and antifibrinolytic activities after its activation into thrombin by the prothrombinase complex. Thrombin acts by activating factors XIII, XI, VIII and V, as well as protein C (PC) and thrombin activatable fibrinolytic inhibitor. It also cleaves fibrinogen to form fibrin. So, the prothrombin gene (*F2*) was widely described as an obvious candidate associated with the risk of VT. It has been identified the prothrombin 20210A mutation (g.20210G>A; rs1799963) in the 3'-UTR region [24-26]. The prevalence of the prothrombin 20210A allele in the general population is 1.7-3.0%, while in VT patients is about 6.2% [18]. Carriers of the 20210A allele is associated with a 3-4 fold increased risk of VT [19], and increased prothrombin levels in plasma. This is probably due to a change in a polyadenylation efficiency of the protein [27], leading to increased thrombin generation, which results in a hypercoagulable state [24]. The mutation also contributes to the regulation of the PC anticoagulant pathway [28]. Carriership of the prothrombin 20210A allele, have an increased risk of recurrences [29], and the presence of other VT risk factors, such as the presence of the FV Leiden [30-34], *PROCR* haplotypes [35] or the ABO blood system [23], modifies their risk.

The mechanism by which prothrombin 20210A increases VT risk via increased prothrombin levels is not fully understood. There is some evidence that prothrombin levels affect the APC-resistance phenotype, but the precise mechanism is not known.

Another SNP located in the intron 13 of the *F2* gene (g.19911A>G; rs3136516), has been associated with increased prothrombin levels [36, 37]. An *in vitro* study [38] demonstrated that the rs3136516 is also functional through its effect on an intronic splicing enhancer motif [18, 25, 36-38].

1.3. Fibrinogen Gene

Fibrinogen is a key component of the haemostatic system, playing a role in both primary and secondary response [39]. Thrombin-catalyzed cleavage of fibrinopeptides A and B converts fibrinogen into fibrin, which spontaneously polymerizes, forming the fibrin clot. The fibrinogen is a disulfide-bonded-dimer molecule consisting of three polypeptides named Aα, Bβ, and γ. The three polypeptides are encoded by separate genes, *FGA*, *FGB*, and *FGG*, respectively, clustered in a region of approximately 50 kb [40]. The *FGG* mRNA transcript is subject to alternative processing and polyadenylation [41].

The main form, the γA chain, consists of 411 amino acids, and results from the use of the polyadenylation signal downstream of exon 10. Whereas, the alternative γ' chain results from the use of an alternative polyadenylation signal in intron 9.

Fibrinogen is a well-established predictor of cardiovascular disease outcomes such as myocardial infarction (MI) [42, 43] stroke, [44] and VT [45, 46]. It is estimated that individual variation in fibrinogen levels is heritable [47, 48], indicating a substantial influence of genetic factors. Several meta-analyses of fibrinogen GWAS studies, conducted in cohorts of European ancestry, identified several genetic variants affecting plasma fibrinogen levels [49, 50]. But, a recent meta-analysis of fibrinogen GWAS studies, based on a 4-fold greater sample size than other meta-analyses (>100000 subjects), identified up to 24 independent signals in 23 loci (of which 15 are new). Clinical outcome analysis of these loci does not support a causal relationship between circulating levels of fibrinogen and coronary artery disease, stroke, or VT [51].

Increased levels of fibrinogen have been proposed to promote fibrin formation, increase platelet aggregation and viscosity, or simply reflect an inflammatory state [52]. Several studies have highlighted the existence of a first-order relationship between fibrinogen concentration and fibrinolysis rate [53], suggesting that increased fibrinogen levels may actually cause thrombosis by slowing fibrinolysis rates [54]. The association between fibrinogen γ′ and VT is controversial.

The first publication on this subject, a case-control study (N=948) from the Leiden Thrombophilia Study (LETS), showed that VT patients have reduced γA/γ' fibrinogen levels and reduced γ' fibrinogen/total fibrinogen ratio compared to healthy controls [46, 55]. There is a significant association between the *FGG*-H2 haplotype, that contains the *FGG* g.10034C>T SNP (rs2066865), and VT [46]. The *FGG*-H2 haplotype is associated with reduced γA/γ' fibrinogen levels and is robustly associated with an increased risk of VT [46]. Individuals with a γ' fibrinogen/total fibrinogen ratio below the 10th percentile, as measured in the control group, had a 2.4-fold increased risk of VT in the LETS. A recent GWAS study demonstrated that the genetic loci associated with γ' fibrinogen levels are all located in or near the fibrinogen gene locus, the strongest association being observed with the *FGG* rs2066865 [56]. However this SNP is in linkage disequilibrium with the *FGA* Thr312Ala (rs6050) variation, that results in hard clots with increased Aα chain cross-linking, larger string diameters, and a lower number of string per unit area [57]. The authors suggested that γ′ fibrinogen was protective against VT due to its antithrombin (AT) activity [58]. It appears that the relationship between γA/γ' fibrinogen level and thrombosis may depend on the type of vascular disease, whereby the γ' chain associates with a prothrombotic risk in arterial disease, but with an antithrombotic effect in VT [46, 59]. It has been proposed that the γ′ chain has a high affinity binding site for active thrombin, and as a result, there is less free thrombin available to cleave its substrates. Therefore, low γ′ fibrinogen levels may cause reduced sequestration of thrombin, a hypercoagulable state and high risk of VT [60]. Binding of the γ′ chain to thrombin allosterically modulates the active site [61]. In addition, this AT activity also inhibits FVIII cleavage [62] and thrombin activation of platelets by limiting PAR1 cleavage [62, 63]. Studies with transgenic mice containing the human fibrinogen thrombin-binding γ′ chain sequence showed a decrease in thrombosis [64].

In contrast, Cheung et al. reported that γ′ fibrinogen levels during the acute phase of pulmonary embolism (PE) were highest [65]. Several studies have suggested that a possible explanation for these results is that, upon binding of thrombin to the γ chain, the cleavage of thrombin´s substrates is changed, such as thrombomodulin (TM) [66], platelet glycoprotein Ib α [67] or

AT [68]. This would potentially allow continued clot formation at the site where fibrin is being deposited, preventing diffusion of thrombin to blood flow and growing clot surface. Further studies will be necessary to definitively address the association between γ′ fibrinogen and VT.

1.4. Natural Anticoagulants of Coagulation and Risk of Thrombosis

The coagulation process is under the control of several inhibitors that limit clot formation near the damaged vessel wall, thus avoiding thrombus propagation. This delicate balance can be interrupted whenever the pro-coagulant activity of one of the coagulation factors is increased or the activity of one of the naturally occurring inhibitors decreases, leading to thrombus formation. Inherited AT, PC, and protein S (PS) deficiencies are rare but strong risk factors for venous thrombosis, although they have moderate or low effect on arterial thrombosis.

1.4.1. Antithrombin Gene

AT belongs to the serpin family of proteins and circulates in plasma acting as one of the most important natural anticoagulant that regulates coagulation by inhibiting procoagulant serine proteases such as thrombin [69, 70], activated (a) FX and FIX [71]. AT acts as suicide inhibitor, forming stable 1:1 enzyme-AT complexes in which the active site of the target proteinase, interacts with the reactive site of the inhibitor.

Based on the circulating antigen level and functional activity of AT, two types of AT deficiency can be distinguished. Type I AT deficiency is defined by a proportional decrease of the AT antigen and activity, whereas type II AT deficiency is characterized by a reduction of the AT activity and normal or almost normal AT antigen levels.

Decreased AT plasma levels have been associated with VT risk in a dose–response manner [72], suggesting that mutations which modulate AT levels variability could also be good candidates for VT risk. Egeberg was the first to identify a genetic risk factor for VT, the AT deficiency, by studying a family with many relatives affected by VT [73].

AT deficiency has been classified as a strong genetic risk factor for VT [74], with a relative thrombotic risk around 10 [19], although it is relatively rare in the general population (0.02%). AT deficiency is transmitted as an autosomal dominant trait, and due to the embryonic lethality of severe AT deficiency, affected individuals are heterozygous [75, 76]. Since the original description [73], more than 227 distinct mutations in the AT gene (*SERPINC1*) have been described 216 of them related to AT deficiency [76, 77], approximately 50-60% of that mutations are missense [76, 78], and most of them reported an association between SNP and AT levels [79] and/or VT risk [12].

A GWAS study with ~900 individuals of the MARTHA project, identified several common SNPs (i.e. with minor allele frequency MAF > 5%) that causes a modified AT plasma levels [80]. However, there isn't any common SNP identified that could explain even 5% of plasma AT variability.

Homozygous AT deficiency is not compatible with life except for few homozygous or hemizygous patients with type II deficiency. Several AT deficiencies type II have been described. the most common being AT Budapest III (p.Leu131Phe) and AT Toyama (p.Arg79Cys) were associated with a soft thrombotic risk [81, 82], and AT Cambridge II (p.Ala416Ser), which is the most prevalent in normal population [83] causing an inefficient inhibition of thrombin [84], increase the potential thrombin generation [85], and a moderately increases the risk of venous and arterial thrombosis [83, 86].

Some family-based studies have evaluated the risk of thrombosis in AT deficient individuals and their relatives [87-89]. However, few studies have investigated the association between the risk of thrombosis in AT deficiency and *SERPINC1* mutations [83, 86, 90]. A recent retrospective cohort study showed that *SERPINC1* missense mutations are associated with a lower risk of VT and tended to have higher risk of arterial thrombosis compared to null mutations (deletions, insertions, nonsense mutations, and splice site mutations) [91].

1.4.2. Protein C Gene

PC is a vitamin k-dependent serine protease that acts as regulator of the coagulation cascade. PC circulates in plasma as a zymogen that is activated by the thrombin/TM complex [92], a reaction that is further enhanced by the endothelial PC receptor (EPCR) [93]. When activated PC (APC) is bound to its cofactor, the protein S (PS), it exerts an antithrombotic effect through proteolysis of the procoagulant FVa and FVIIIa, limiting the coagulation cascade and fibrin formation [94, 95]. Moreover, APC also exerts anti-inflammatory and cytoprotective activities, which includes antiapoptotic activity, neurological and endothelial barrier protection, and modulation of gene expression [96]. These activities require binding of APC to EPCR and activation of the thrombin receptor PAR1 to initialize a cascade of cell signaling [97].

PC was described as a thrombotic risk factor in 1981, when Griffin et al. described a heterozygous PC deficiency in a family with a history of recurrent VT. The deficiency in homozygosis was described in 1984 by Seligsohn et al. [98] and Estellés et al. [92] in a newborn with disseminated intravascular coagulation and purpura fulminans within hours of birth.

There are two types of PC deficiencies: type I which is characterized by the reduction of antigen and functional levels, and type II, characterized by the presence of normal antigen levels and a reduction in the anticoagulant activity, which implies the presence of abnormal circulating PC molecules.

In the general population, low levels of circulating PC and APC is associated with an increased risk of VT [99, 100]. PC deficiency is usually due to privative mutations in the PC gene (*PROC*) and occurs in 1/ 250-500 of the adult population [19]. The thrombotic risk associated with heterozygous PC deficiency is approximately 8 fold, compared with individuals without any deficiency [19].

It is important to mention that the detection of both types of PC deficiencies is usually tested by measuring circulating PC levels and the functional activity of PC by chromogenic substrates. Thus, there are some undetected mutations that provide changes in substrate recognition sites, cofactor or membrane binding sites, which result in normal APC levels but reduced activity.

Several SNPs (including rs1799810, rs2069910, and rs2069915) located in the promoter of *PROC* mildly influence PC plasma levels [101-103], and also other SNPs located in other locus [104] (i.e. *PROCR and GCKR* loci [105]) will influence the plasma levels of PC.

Currently, there are more than 272 different mutations described in *PROC* and related to PC deficiency in the Human Gene Mutation Database (http://www.hgmd.cf.ac.uk).

Several SNPs located in the promoter of the *PROC* gene have been shown to mildly influence the PC plasma levels [101-103]. A study in a Dutch population showed that the most frequent missense mutations were found in the Gln132 and Arg230 residues, leading to type I PC deficiency [106]. In French population, some studies showed that the most frequent type I mutations were in the Arg178 and Pro168 residues [107, 108]. Regarding type II PC deficiency, the change Arg to Gln in the residue 229, in a family with a history of VT [109].

Structure-function studies showed that the 229Gln mutation alters the activation of PC by the thrombin-TM complex [110, 111], which can explain the reduced biological activity of this PC variant, although PC plasma levels and enzymatic capacity remain unaltered.

1.4.3. Protein S Gene

PS is a 69 kD vitamin K-dependent plasma glycoprotein that acts as a non-enzymatic cofactor of APC and tissue factor pathway inhibitor [112-115].

PS circulates at a concentration of approximately 350 nM, which 40% is free and 60% forms inactive complexes with C4b-binding protein [116]. Only the free PS fraction has APC cofactor activity. PS deficiency is a risk factor for VT that affects approximately 5% of thrombophilic patients and 1–2% of consecutive patients with a first VT [16, 117]. Assessment of the thrombotic risk caused by PS deficiency is difficult due to the lack of sufficiently large studies examining its prevalence in the general population [118-123]. Although one large prospective case–control study failed to find an association between PS deficiency and venous thrombosis [118, 121], a 2.4 fold increased risk of thrombosis has been reported among PS deficient patients, while family-based studies have reported a 5–8.5 fold higher risk of thrombosis amongst affected relatives of PS deficient patients when compared with unaffected relatives [119, 120]. Three types of PS deficiency have been described: type I (decreased levels of both total and free PS antigen), type II (decreased APC cofactor activity but normal total and free PS antigen levels), and type III (decreased levels of free PS antigen levels only) [16, 117, 124]. Diagnosis of PS deficiency is complicated because of the inter- and intra-individual variation in plasma PS levels, and by the overlap in levels between unaffected individuals and those having heterozygous deficiencies. Several factors including age, sex, hormonal state, pregnancy, liver disease and inflammation can influence plasma PS levels, further complicating diagnosis [125-128]. The first VT patients with PS deficiency were described by Comp et al. in 1984 [129, 130]. Hereditary PS deficiency is due to rare and privative mutations within PS gene (*PROS1*). More than 234 mutations in *PROS1* have been described, the majority missense or nonsense mutations (http://www.hgmd.cf.ac.uk) [124, 131, 132], 210 of them related with PS deficiency. Sequencing of exons and splicing junctions of *PROS1* has lead to the identification of a mutation in approximately 50% of families with PS deficiency [131]. Moreover, large deletions and insertions in *PROS1* are present in approximately 30% of the point mutation-negative families [133-135]. Bertina et al. in 1990 [136] described the Heerlen polymorphism, which causes a Ser460Pro substitution in the mature PS and is characterized by the presence of a PS molecule in plasma that has a lower molecular weight than normal PS. The biological significance of the Heerlen mutation is unclear. In one study, the allele was present in 1/192 (0.52%) chromosomes tested in a control population compared to 16/1182 (0.68%) chromosomes in consecutive VT patients [136]. However, in another study the Heerlen allele was shown to be more frequent among patients with type III PS deficiency than those with type I deficiency [137].

In addition, the Heerlen variant produces changes in the binding stoichiometry to C4BP-b that could result in a reduction in free PS levels.

In the MARTHA [80] and GAIT GWAS studies [138] common SNPs associated with PS levels were identified. These two studies failed to detect robust associations despite some suggestive elements in favor of an association of *DNAJC6* SNPs with free PS levels [138].

1.5. ABO Locus

High plasma levels of von Willebrand factor (vWF) and FVIII are well-established risk factor for VT [139]. Overall, approximately 70% of the variation in plasma levels of vWF and FVIII is genetically determined, with 30% explained by the individual ABO blood group [140]. Notably, vWF and FVIII levels are approximately 25% higher in individuals who have a non O-blood group [141-144]. The frequency of non-O blood group in patients with deep vein thrombosis (DVT) [143, 144] or VT [145-147] was significantly higher compared to the healthy blood donors [142]. Moreover, non-O individuals had higher concentrations of both factor VIII and VWF as compared to those group O subjects [142, 145, 146]. In addition, the risk was increased in non-O individuals carrying other inherited thrombophilic defects, such as FVL, prothrombin 20210A mutation, AT, PC and PS deficiencies [23, 142, 144, 146, 147].

Jick et al. [148] were the first to report that non-O blood group was associated with increased risk of VT. Recent studies [5, 8, 147, 149] have clarified this association and demonstrated that B and A1 blood groups had higher VT risk than O and A2 blood groups.

In addition, O and A2 groups can be genetically determined by the rs817 6719 and rs8176750 SNPs, and were consistently found at a lower frequency in VT patients than in controls in the three GWAS reported so far on VT [5, 8, 149, 150].

In depth analysis of the ABO locus, has recently identified several intronic and 3'UTR SNPs which evidenced that the association between VT and the ABO blood group could be independent of the rs8176750 and rs8176719 SNPs [149, 151]. All these studies emphasized the known complexity of the link between ABO locus and VT risk.

The mechanism by which ABO blood group is believed to contribute to VT risk is through modifications of VWF and FVIII levels in plasma, likely by affecting VWF glycosylation and thus its proteolysis and clearance [152, 153].

However, ABO blood groups remain significantly associated with VT even after adjustment for FVIII or vWF levels in cardiovascular diseases [146, 154].

This suggests that ABO may affect cardiovascular risk by other means than solely modifications of FVIII and vWF molecules.

First, although traditionally regarded as red blood cell antigen, ABO antigens are also expressed on various other tissues including platelets, the vascular endothelium, and epithelial surfaces [152].

Second, the ABO locus was found associated with plasma levels of soluble intercellular adhesion molecule-1, P-selectin, and E-selectin [155], three intermediate phenotypes of cardiovascular risk.

2. Emerging Genetic Risk Factors for Thrombosis

2.1. Von Willebrand Factor Gene

As previously mentioned, ABO blood group affects vWF glycosylation leading to increased VT risk [152, 153]. Moreover, genetic variation in the vWF gene (*VWF*) can also influence the risk of VT.

The *VWF* rs1063856 SNP, resulting in a Thr789Ala substitution in exon 18, is associated with increased vWF levels and VT risk (OR ~ 1.15) [156]. A meta-analysis of several GWAS datasets conducted under the CHARGE consortium [157] identified 6 novel loci modulating vWF plasma levels, CLEC4M, STX2, TC2N, STXBP5, SCARA5, and STAB 2 among which the latter three also influenced FVIII levels.

Therefore, these loci are natural candidates for VT risk. However none of the vWF-associated SNPs at the CLEC4M, STX2, and SCARA5 have been found so far associated with VT risk.

Conversely, TAB 2 [150, 158], TC2N [6], and STXBP5 [157] SNPs have been observed associated with VT risk but there is yet no evidence for a functional role of the STAB 2 and TC2N VT-associated SNPs.

The missense rs1039084 STXBP5 SNP (Asn436Ser) could be functional. Evidence for a role of STXBP5 in the regulation of vWF has been recently reinforced by the finding that STXBP5 SNPs were associated with a bleeding phenotype in women with type 1 von Willebrand disease [159].

2.2. Factor XI Gene

Meijers et al. [160] reported that high FXI levels were associated with increased risk of VT. FXI circulates as a zymogen as a complex with high molecular weight kininogen (HMWK) [161] and contributes to haemostasis by activating FIX. FXI can be activated by four biologically relevant proteases: FXIIa, FXIa, thrombin, and meizothrombin. The most relevant *in vivo* pathway for plasma FXI activation seems to be the feedback activation by thrombin [162]. Later, in 2007, several SNPs, including rs2036914, rs3822057 and rs2289252, at the *F11* locus were reported to be associated with the risk of VT (with OR ~1.35) through modulation of FXI plasma levels [12, 20, 163].

2.3. Glicoprotein 6 Gene

The glycoprotein 6 gene (*GP6*) is the first VT-associated locus that lies outside the standard coagulation cascade. It was identified through a large-scale association study, focusing mainly on non-synonymous polymorphisms [12]. *GP6* encodes the receptor glycoprotein VI that has a major role in collagen induced signalling.

It is a crucial platelet membrane glycoprotein, for adequate platelet activation, adhesion and aggregation. The *G6P* rs1613662 (Ser219Pro) SNP, was associated with a 15% increased risk of VT [8, 164]. Although the precise mechanism is unknown, the Ser219Pro change modified the collagen receptor GPVI, and produced a reduction in the collagen-induced platelet activation in a dose-dependent manner [165]. The identification of *GP6* as a VT-associated locus is striking as it indicates that platelets play a determining role in VT although they have historically been ignored in this pathological setting. Activated platelets are important catalysts of both intrinsic and extrinsic thrombin generation and, therefore, fibrin deposition [166]. Kotuličová D et al.

2012 studied the genetic variability of *GP6* in patients with platelet hyperaggregability phenotype, known as sticky platelet syndrome (SPS) and manifesting as DVT, and/or pulmonary embolism. A significant association between 1613662-G [$P < 0.05$, odds ratio (OR) 2.087, confidence interval (CI) 1.049-4.148], and VTE was found in patients with SPS. They also found association between VTE and another GP6 rs1654419 SNP ($P<0.05$, OR=2.161, CI 95%=1.020-4.577), in patients with SPS. However, there was not found association between the studied GP6 genotypes and the severity of VTE (pulmonary embolism vs. DVT) was found [167].

2.4. Protein C System and Risk of Thrombosis

As previously mentioned the PC system plays a crucial role in the regulation of blood coagulation in humans.

APC generation depends on the precise coupling, on the surface of endothelial cells, of thrombin and PC to their respective receptors, TM and EPCR. Any change in the efficiency of this coupling may cause altered APC generation and a modification in the risk of thrombosis. In fact, several mutations have been reported in *PROCR* or TM gene (*THBD*), some of them associated with the risk of thrombosis.

2.4.1. EPCR Gene

EPCR is a 46-kD type I transmembrane protein, constitutively expressed on the luminal surface of the endothelial cells of large vessels, and is structurally similar to the major histocompatibility class 1/CD1 family proteins involved in the immune and inflammation responses [168]. Thus, it expression had been reduced by inflammatory stimuli, like tumor necrosis factor-α, or an atherosclerotic setting [168, 169]. EPCR is also expressed in the surface of other cell types [170-182], which suggests the role of EPCR in other disorders. In fact, Animal experiments have demonstrated the importance of EPCR in normal embryonic development, in *PROCR* knockout mice, fibrin deposition in trophoblast giant cells results in thrombosis at the maternal-embryonic interface [183].

A soluble form of EPCR (sEPCR) also circulates in the plasma. By limiting APC generation and function, elevated levels of sEPCR may exert procoagulant and proinflammatory effects; in 2 case-control studies [35, 184] elevated levels of sEPCR were associated with increased risk of VT. Likewise, a small family study found a higher occurrence of VT in those with above normal values of sEPCR compared with those with normal levels [185].

Functional polymorphisms in the *PROCR* gene may increase/decrease the risk of thrombosis, especially in carriers of other prothrombotic mutations, as VT is a multifactorial disease [186, 187]. Rare point mutations within the gene [188] and its promoter region [189] have been described, but their effect on thrombosis and gene expression remain unknown given its low population frequency [190]. The first *PROCR* gene mutation described was a 23bp insertion in exon 3, at position 4031 [191], and results in a STOP codon downstream from the insertion point [188]. Expression studies in mammalian cells showed that the truncated protein is not localized on the cell surface, can not be secreted in the culture medium, and does not bind APC, suggesting that the insertion is a risk factor for arterial and venous thrombosis. However, given its low population frequency (<1%) [192, 193], statistical analysis did not reveal a significant association between the mutation and the risk of thrombosis [188, 191, 192, 194-196].

Franchi et al. [197] described a mutation in the promoter region of the *PROCR* gene, g.(-318)T>G substitution, present in 1/95 women with late fetal loss and in 0/236 controls. Biguzzi et al. [189] reported four point mutations in the *PROCR* gene promoter.

However, they were rare in patients with VT or MI, and the *in vitro* characterization did not reveal any decreased activity of the reporter gene in basal conditions. Hermida et al. identified a heterozygous C to T variation at position 2769, which predicts a substitution of Arg to Cys at position 98 in the mature protein [198]. However, its low population prevalence and the *in vitro* expression and characterization of this mutation suggested no role of this mutation in VT [198].

Simmonds and Lane [199] reported the organization and nucleotide sequence of the human *PROCR* and suggested two potential polymorphic sites, the g.2532T>C substitution in intron 1 and the g.4600A>G substitution in exon 4 that predicts a Ser219Gly change.

In the last years, up to four haplotypes of *PROCR* have been reported [184, 200, 201]: H1, H2, H3 and H4, three of which contain one or more haplotype-specific SNPs, while H2 contains the common allele of each SNP.

The *PROCR* H1 haplotype tagged by the rare allele of g.4678G>C (rs9574), has been associated with increased circulating APC levels [202] and a reduced risk of VT in 2 independent studies (OR = 0.59, 95% CI=0.41–0.84) [201, 203]. H1 also reduced the risk of thrombosis in carriers of FV Leiden (OR=0.31; 95%CI=0.16–0.83) [22].

In patients with the FV Leiden mutation, the mean age at the first thrombosis was significantly higher in propositi carrying the H1H1 genotype than in non-carriers of the H1 haplotype. In addition, the probability of being free of thrombosis at age 40 was significantly higher in propositi carriers of the H1H1 genotype than in the non carriers ($P<0.001$). In contrast, two other groups found no association of the H1 haplotype with the risk of thrombosis [200] or a slight reduction of the risk [184].

A possible explanation for the protective effect of the *PROCR* H1 haplotype against VT, both in patients with no thrombophilic mutations and in carriers of FV Leiden, would be its association with increased APC levels. It has been described that a low level of APC in plasma is a strong, prevalent, independent risk factor for VT [100, 204].

In fact, reduced APC levels increased the risk of VT 4.7-fold, and a preliminary familial study revealed that in some instances the low APC phenotype is hereditary.

Presently it is unknown which SNP in EPCR H1 is responsible for the reported protective effect.

The H1 haplotype contains 10 specific alleles, the 1451T (rs2069943), 1541A (rs2069944), 1880C (rs2069945), 2532C (rs2069948), 2897A (rs945 960), 3424C (rs871480), 3997C (rs2069952), 4678C (rs9574), 5632G (rs1415 773), and 5663A (rs1415774). Therefore, any of these nucleotides may be responsible for the observed association of the *PROCR* H1 haplotype with increased levels of plasma APC and reduced risk of VT. Further studies are required to identify which polymorphism/s is/are responsible for the observed associations. The *PROCR* H3 haplotype tagged by the rare allele of g.4600A>G (rs867186), is associated with increased plasma levels of sEPCR [35, 184, 200, 201, 205-208] and increase VT risk [105, 200, 209].

Regarding the SNPs that comprise the *PROCR* H3 haplotype, the 4600G allele is the more obvious candidate responsible for the association of *PROCR* H3 haplotype with increased sEPCR levels, in view of the fact that the cleavage of the EPCR anchored in the endothelial cell membrane to generate sEPCR occurs within the region of the protein encoded by exon 4, near the 4600 position. The 4600G variant predicts a conformational change in the protein due to the Ser 219 to Gly substitution, which could render an EPCR more susceptible to cleavage by metalloprotease such as ADAM17 [200, 201]. This hypothesis has been supported by two independent studies [206, 210].

Other mechanism that could link the H3 haplotype and high levels of sEPCR is the alternative splicing reported by Saposnik et al. [211]. In both cases, the increased shedding of EPCR could reduce the amount of EPCR at the endothelial surface and explain the increased Vt risk associated with H3. In favor of this argument is the fact that inducing EPCR shedding in cells bearing the H3 haplotype notably reduced their hability to sustain PC activation as compared with non-H3 cells [210].

Studies looking for genetic determinants for PC levels have shown that the *PROCR* H3 is associated with higher plasma PC levels [103, 105]. Additionally, the H3 haplotype has also been associated with higher levels of FVII [157, 212], which could also explain the increased VT risk associated to this haplotype. One study demonstrated that *PROCR* H3 also increases the risk of VT in carriers of the prothrombin 20210A mutation, probably due to its association with increased sEPCR levels, and that H3 carriers experienced the first VT episode at a young age [35].

Nevertheless, the molecular mechanism by which the increased sEPCR levels observed in individuals bearing the H3 haplotype could increase the risk of venous thrombosis remains to be determined.

It has been described that an increased physiological sEPCR concentration result in decreased PC activation and inhibition of generated APC [200].

Finally, *PROCR* H4 haplotype was reported to be associated with a slight increase in the risk of VT [184], although no further studies have confirmed these results.

2.4.2. Thrombomodulin Gene

TM is an endothelial cell membrane protein that acts as a receptor for thrombin in the activation of PC. TM is also independently involved in cytoprotective responses [213-216]. Studies in animal models suggest that TM deficiency is associated with a prethrombotic state [217-219].

Heterogeneous soluble forms of TM (sTM) circulate in plasma [220] and their levels are increased in several clinical conditions [221]. Some of these soluble forms might have anticoagulant activity [222]. According to the assay used for the measurements, range from 2.7 to 5.4 ng/ml [223] or from 25 to 65 ng/ml [224].

Genetic studies have identified a number of mutations and polymorphisms in the *THBD* gene, but no clear association with venous or arterial thrombosis has been found [225]. A common SNP in the coding region of *THBD* (c.1418 C>T; rs1042579), which results in the replacement of Ala455 by Val, has been described [226]. This dimorphism is located in the TM region responsible for thrombin binding and PC activation, suggesting a potential role in the modulation of TM function.

However, its association with venous [226-230] and arterial thrombosis [231-233] is not consistent.

Several studies have investigated the association between the *THBD* c.14 18C>T polymorphism and venous and arterial thrombosis, with conflicting results. Some studies did not find an association between the polymorphism and the risk of VT [229, 230]. Others have described a lower risk of VT in blacks carrying the *THBD* 1418T allele [229] or a protective effect for the T allele in arterial thrombosis [232], whereas others reported a higher risk or VT in the presence of the *THBD* 1418T allele in Japanese population [234] or an increased risk of coronary heart disease associated with the presence of the *THBD* 1418T allele in Caucasians [235] and black population [233].

An explanation for these discrepancies may lie in differences in study designs and patient populations, age and small sample sizes.

A recent large case-control study [236], in Caucasians, provided new data on the age dependent association between the presence of the *THBD* 1418T allele and a lower VT risk.

Moreover, additional analysis in this study, showed that human umbilical vein endothelial cells (HUVEC) carrying the *THBD* 1418T allele (Val455), had lower sTM levels in culture supernatant, increased membrane–bound TM, and increased cellular TM activity, defined as the thrombin-mediated PC activation on intact HUVEC, whereas the *THBD* mRNA level was similar in carriers and non-carriers. The mechanism by which the *THBD* 1418T allele protects against VT is not clear.

One explanation could be that the Val455 form has higher cofactor activity for PC activation. However, recombinant Val455 and Ala455, produced by Cos-1 cells, were found equally active in PC activation [237]. Another explanation could be that the *THBD* 1418T allele is associated with increased membrane-bound TM, resulting in increased PC activation, but no significant differences in *THBD* mRNA levels according to the *THBD* c.1418 C>T polymorphism in HUVEC cell studies were found [236]. Soluble TM represents cleaved forms of membrane-bound TM with loss of part of the serine–threonine rich region, the transmembrane domain, and the cytoplasmic tail [238], and the TM 455Ala residue is located not far from the presumed cleavage site.

So it is possible that the membrane-bound TM carrying the 455Val (1418T allele) might be more stable and less prone to shedding and may induce a protection from TM cleavage by proteases, which will result in higher PC activation rate and a lower risk of VT. Regarding to the levels of sTM, the association is controversial.

It has been reported that increased levels of sTM are associated with higher VT risk, and this association was, at least in part, independent of the *THBD* c.1418C>T polymorphism [236].

In contrast, increased sTM levels have also been reported in patients with recurrent VT [239], and other studies did not find any association between sTM and risk of VT [229].

Alternatively, the observed association between the *THBD* c.1418C>T polymorphism and the risk of VT could be attributed to another polymorphism in tight linkage disequilibrium with c.1418C>T.

In fact, some studies observed complete linkage disequilibrium ($r2$=0.98) between the c.1418C>T and c.2729 A>C (rs3176123) polymorphisms, and a moderate linkage disequilibrium between the c.1418C>T and c.–1208-1209del TT ($r2$=0.27) [236, 240].

2.5. Emerging Genes

A new estimate of the genetic variance associated with VT susceptibility was also derived using several GWAS and meta-analysis [6-12], conducted on thousands of individuals.

These emerging genes were robustly associated with VT, although, further analyses in case-control studies are necessary to confirm their association.

Results from GWAS and gene expression analyses [11] identified the *C4 BPA/C4BPB* genes as new susceptibility loci for VT with unknown PS-independent mechanism. *C4BPA* and *C4BPB* genes coding for the α- and β-chains of the C4b-BP, a heterodimeric molecule existing in three different isoforms: $\alpha7\beta1$, $\alpha6\beta1$, and $\alpha7\beta0$. The rs3813948-C allele was found associated with increased levels of both $\alpha7\beta0$ and *C4BPA* expression and increased risk of VT in two French case–control studies [11].

This SNP was not associated with PS levels, this emphasizes the previously raised possibility that C4b-BP can be independently active in the coagulation pathway [241].

Moreover, C4b-BP also belongs to complement inactivate proteins which are thought to be involved in immune response and inflammation, and this could favor a role of inflammation in VT-related mechanisms [242]. Another association was observed for the *SERPINF2* rs8074026. *SERPINF2* is an obvious candidate for VT as it codes for a serpine protease inhibitor that acts as plasmin inhibitor.

However, no trend for association was observed in the replication study. Two GWAS analyses identified the *STAB2* rs1593812 / rs4981021 haplo-type to increase the risk of VT [158]. *STAB2* encodes for stabilin-2.

HIVEP1 encodes a protein that participates in the transcriptional regulation of inflammatory target genes. A GWAS analyses showed that *HIV EP1* rs169713 SNP increase VT risk [10] and the rs169715/ rs2228220 haplo-type (r2 = 0.09) also increase the VT risk, but with an additive effect [150]. Following the findings of a GWAS on aPTT levels [243], a candidate bio-marker for VT it has been recently suggested, the *KNG1* gene, encoding the HK protein. HK plays an important role in blood coagulation bringing near prekallikrein, FXI and FXII [244].

Later, another study [245], showed that the *KNG1* rs710446 (p.Ile581Thr) SNP was also associated with increased VT.

More recently, the GAIT study [246] has shown that the rs710446 SNP was also associated with plasma FXI concentration.

3. Final Remarks

This chapter summarizes the main current information on the role of genetic risk factors for venous thrombosis. Pathogenesis of thrombosis has to be considered within a multifaceted perspective, as confirmed by the amount of epidemiological data on both genetic and environmental thrombotic risk factors.

Nevertheless, a significant proportion of thrombotic episodes, especially among young individuals, occur without a plausible explanation. On the other hand, many thrombosis patients have more than one predisposing genetic and/ or environmental risk factor, and there is convincing evidence that risk increases in proportion to the number of predisposing factors.

Traditional thrombotic risk factors, environmentals, acquired and genetics, play a role in VT, but fail to fully explain the pathology. Further basic and clinical research is needed to reach a correct identification of new factors associated with VT and/or arterial thrombosis, in order to assess the individual risk of thrombosis and promote more targeted prophylactic and therapeutic options.

Acknowledgments

Funding sources: This work was supported by the PN de I+D+I 2008-20011 of Instituto de Salud Carlos III-Fondo de Investigación Sanitaria and FEDER (PI12/00027 and Red Temática de Investigación RIC RD12/0042/0029), Conselleria de Educación-Generalitat Valenciana (Prometeo/2011/027), and Fundación para la Investigación del Hospital Universitario La Fe (2007-0185), Spain. Pilar Medina is a Miguel Servet Researcher (ISCIII CP09/000 65).

References

[1] White, R. H., The epidemiology of venous thromboembolism. *Circulation* 2003, 107, I4-8.

[2] Prandoni, P., Bernardi, E., Marchiori, A., Lensing, A. W., Prins, M. H., Villalta, S., Bagatella, P., Sartor, D., Piccioli, A., Simioni, P., Pagnan, A., Girolami, A., The long term clinical course of acute deep vein thrombosis of the arm: prospective cohort study. *BMJ* 2004, 329, 484-5.

[3] Coombes, R., Venous thromboembolism caused 25,000 deaths a year, say MPs. *BMJ* 2005, 330, 559.

[4] Heit, J. A., The epidemiology of venous thromboembolism in the community. *Arterioscler. Thromb. Vasc. Biol.* 2008, 28, 370-2.

[5] Morange, P. E., Trégouët, D. A., Current knowledge on the genetics of incident venous thrombosis. *J. Thromb. Haemost.* 2013, 11 Suppl. 1, 111-21.

[6] Morange, P. E., Saut, N., Antoni, G., Emmerich, J., Trégouët, D. A., Impact on venous thrombosis risk of newly discovered gene variants associated with FVIII and VWF plasma levels. *J. Thromb. Haemost.* 2011, 9, 229-31.

[7] Souto, J. C., Almasy, L., Borrell, M., Blanco-Vaca, F., Mateo, J., Soria, J. M., Coll, I., Felices, R., Stone, W., Fontcuberta, J., Blangero, J., Genetic susceptibility to thrombosis and its relationship to physiological risk factors: the GAIT study. Genetic Analysis of Idiopathic Thrombophilia. *Am. J. Hum. Genet.* 2000, 67, 1452-9.

[8] Trégouët, D. A., Heath, S., Saut, N., Biron-Andreani, C., Schved, J. F., Pernod, G., Galan, P., Drouet, L., Zelenika, D., Juhan-Vague, I., Alessi, M. C., Tiret, L., Lathrop, M., Emmerich, J., Morange, P. E., Common

susceptibility alleles are unlikely to contribute as strongly as the FV and ABO loci to VTE risk: results from a GWAS approach. *Blood* 2009, 113, 5298-303.

[9] Rosendaal, F. R., Reitsma, P. H., Genetics of venous thrombosis. *J. Thromb. Haemost.* 2009, 7 Suppl. 1, 301-4.

[10] Morange, P. E., Bezemer, I., Saut, N., Bare, L., Burgos, G., Brocheton, J., Durand, H., Biron-Andreani, C., Schved, J. F., Pernod, G., Galan, P., Drouet, L., Zelenika, D., Germain, M., Nicaud, V., Heath, S., Ninio, E., Delluc, A., Münzel, T., Zeller, T., Brand-Herrmann, S. M., Alessi, M. C., Tiret, L., Lathrop, M., Cambien, F., Blankenberg, S., Emmerich, J., Trégouët, D. A., Rosendaal, F. R., A follow-up study of a genome-wide association scan identifies a susceptibility locus for venous thrombosis on chromosome 6p24.1. *Am. J. Hum. Genet.* 2010, 86, 592-5.

[11] Buil, A., Trégouët, D. A., Souto, J. C., Saut, N., Germain, M., Rotival, M., Tiret, L., Cambien, F., Lathrop, M., Zeller, T., Alessi, M. C., Rodriguez de Cordoba, S., Münzel, T., Wild, P., Fontcuberta, J., Gagnon, F., Emmerich, J., Almasy, L., Blankenberg, S., Soria, J. M., Morange, P. E., C4BPB/C4BPA is a new susceptibility locus for venous thrombosis with unknown protein S-independent mechanism: results from genome-wide association and gene expression analyses followed by case-control studies. *Blood* 2010, 115, 4644-50.

[12] Bezemer, I. D., Bare, L. A., Doggen, C. J., Arellano, A. R., Tong, C., Rowland, C. M., Catanese, J., Young, B. A., Reitsma, P. H., Devlin, J. J., Rosendaal, F. R., Gene variants associated with deep vein thrombosis. *JAMA* 2008, 299, 1306-14.

[13] Dahlbäck, B., Carlsson, M., Svensson, P. J., Familial thrombophilia due to a previously unrecognized mechanism characterized by poor anticoagulant response to activated protein C: prediction of a cofactor to activated protein C. *Proc. Natl. Acad. Sci. US* 1993, 90, 1004-8.

[14] Bertina, R. M., Koeleman, B. P., Koster, T., Rosendaal, F. R., Dirven, R. J., de Ronde, H., van der Velden, P. A., Reitsma, P. H., Mutation in blood coagulation factor V associated with resistance to activated protein C. *Nature* 1994, 369, 64-7.

[15] De Stefano, V., Rossi, E., Paciaroni, K., Leone, G., Screening for inherited thrombophilia: indications and therapeutic implications. *Haematologica* 2002, 87, 1095-108.

[16] Lane, D. A., Mannucci, P. M., Bauer, K. A., Bertina, R. M., Bochkov, N. P., Boulyjenkov, V., Chandy, M., Dahlbäck, B., Ginter, E. K.,

Miletich, J. P., Rosendaal, F. R., Seligsohn, U., Inherited thrombophilia: Part 1. *Thromb. Haemost.* 1996, 76, 651-62.

[17] Svensson, P. J., Dahlbäck, B., Resistance to activated protein C as a basis for venous thrombosis. *N. Engl. J. Med.* 1994, 330, 517-22.

[18] Previtali, E., Bucciarelli, P., Passamonti, S. M., Martinelli, I., Risk factors for venous and arterial thrombosis. *Blood Transfus.* 2011, 9, 120-38.

[19] Seligsohn, U., Lubetsky, A., Genetic susceptibility to venous thrombosis. *N. Engl. J. Med.* 2001, 344, 1222-31.

[20] Smith, N. L., Hindorff, L. A., Heckbert, S. R., Lemaitre, R. N., Marciante, K. D., Rice, K., Lumley, T., Bis, J. C., Wiggins, K. L., Rosendaal, F. R., Psaty, B. M., Association of genetic variations with nonfatal venous thrombosis in postmenopausal women. *JAMA* 2007, 297, 489-98.

[21] Bezemer, I. D., Bare, L. A., Arellano, A. R., Reitsma, P. H., Rosendaal, F. R., Updated analysis of gene variants associated with deep vein thrombosis. *JAMA* 2010, 303, 421-2.

[22] Medina, P., Navarro, S., Estellés, A., Vayá, A., Bertina, R. M., España, F., Influence of the 4600A/G and 4678G/C polymorphisms in the endothelial protein C receptor (EPCR) gene on the risk of venous thromboembolism in carriers of factor V Leiden. *Thromb. Haemost.* 2005, 94, 389-94.

[23] Sode, B. F., Allin, K. H., Dahl, M., Gyntelberg, F., Nordestgaard, B. G., Risk of venous thromboembolism and myocardial infarction associated with factor V Leiden and prothrombin mutations and blood type. *CMAJ* 2013, 185, E229-37.

[24] Poort, S. R., Rosendaal, F. R., Reitsma, P. H., Bertina, R. M., A common genetic variation in the 3'-untranslated region of the prothrombin gene is associated with elevated plasma prothrombin levels and an increase in venous thrombosis. *Blood* 1996, 88, 3698-703.

[25] Van der Putten, H. H., Bertina, R. M., Vos, H. L., Is the prothrombin 19911A>G polymorphism a functional noncoding variant? *Blood* 2005, 105, 2995; author reply 2995-6.

[26] Van der Putten, H. H., Spaargaren-van Riel, C. C., Bertina, R. M., Vos, H. L., Functional analysis of two prothrombin 3'-untranslated region variants: the C20209T variant, mainly found among African-Americans, and the C20209A variant. *J. Thromb. Haemost.* 2006, 4, 2285-7; author reply 2288-9.

[27] Ceelie, H., Spaargaren-van Riel, C. C., Bertina, R. M., Vos, H. L., G20210A is a functional mutation in the prothrombin gene; effect on protein levels and 3'-end formation. *J.Thromb. Haemost.* 2004, 2, 119-27.

[28] Castoldi, E., Rosing, J., APC resistance: biological basis and acquired influences. *J. Thromb. Haemost.* 2010, 8, 445-53.

[29] Marchiori, A., Mosena, L., Prins, M. H., Prandoni, P., The risk of recurrent venous thromboembolism among heterozygous carriers of factor V Leiden or prothrombin G20210A mutation. A systematic review of prospective studies. *Haematologica* 2007, 92, 1107-14.

[30] Tirado, I., Mateo, J., Soria, J. M., Oliver, A., Borrell, M., Coll, I., Vallvé, C., Souto, J. C., Martínez-Sánchez, E., Fontcuberta, J., Contribution of prothrombin 20210A allele and factor V Leiden mutation to thrombosis risk in thrombophilic families with other hemostatic deficiencies. *Haematologica* 2001, 86, 1200-8.

[31] Emmerich, J., Rosendaal, F. R., Cattaneo, M., Margaglione, M., De Stefano, V., Cumming, T., Arruda, V., Hillarp, A., Reny, J. L., Combined effect of factor V Leiden and prothrombin 20210A on the risk of venous thromboembolism--pooled analysis of 8 case-control studies including 2310 cases and 3204 controls. Study Group for Pooled-Analysis in Venous Thromboembolism. *Thromb. Haemost.* 2001, 86, 809-16.

[32] Martinelli, I., Taioli, E., Bucciarelli, P., Akhavan, S., Mannucci, P. M., Interaction between the G20210A mutation of the prothrombin gene and oral contraceptive use in deep vein thrombosis. *Arterioscler. Thromb. Vasc. Biol.* 1999, 19, 700-3.

[33] Van Rooden, C. J., Rosendaal, F. R., Meinders, A. E., Van Oostayen, J. A., Van Der Meer, F. J., Huisman, M. V., The contribution of factor V Leiden and prothrombin G20210A mutation to the risk of central venous catheter-related thrombosis. *Haematologica* 2004, 89, 201-6.

[34] Gisslinger, H., Müllner, M., Pabinger, I., Heis-Vahidi-Fard, N., Gisslinger, B., Brichta, A., Bachleitner-Hofmann, T., Mannhalter, C., Mutation of the prothrombin gene and thrombotic events in patients with polycythemia vera or essential thrombocythemia: a cohort study. *Haematologica* 2005, 90, 408-10.

[35] Navarro, S., Medina, P., Mira, Y., Estellés, A., Villa, P., Ferrando, F., Vayá, A., Bertina, R. M., España, F., Haplotypes of the EPCR gene, prothrombin levels, and the risk of venous thrombosis in carriers of the prothrombin G20210A mutation. *Haematologica* 2008, 93, 885-91.

[36] Chinthammitr, Y., Vos, H. L., Rosendaal, F. R., Doggen, C. J., The association of prothrombin A19911G polymorphism with plasma prothrombin activity and venous thrombosis: results of the MEGA study, a large population-based case-control study. *J. Thromb. Haemost.* 2006, 4, 2587-92.

[37] Martinelli, I., Battaglioli, T., Tosetto, A., Legnani, C., Sottile, L., Ghiotto, R., Mannucci, P. M., Prothrombin A19911G polymorphism and the risk of venous thromboembolism. *J. Thromb. Haemost.* 2006, 4, 2582-6.

[38] Von Ahsen, N., Oellerich, M., The intronic prothrombin 19911A>G polymorphism influences splicing efficiency and modulates effects of the 20210G>A polymorphism on mRNA amount and expression in a stable reporter gene assay system. *Blood* 2004, 103, 586-93.

[39] Weisel, J. W., Fibrinogen and fibrin. *Adv. Protein Chem.* 2005, 70, 247-99.

[40] Kant, J. A., Fornace, A. J., Saxe, D., Simon, M. I., McBride, O. W., Crabtree, G. R., Evolution and organization of the fibrinogen locus on chromosome 4: gene duplication accompanied by transposition and inversion. *Proc. Natl. Acad. Sci. US* 1985, 82, 2344-8.

[41] Chung, D. W., Davie, E. W., gamma and gamma' chains of human fibrinogen are produced by alternative mRNA processing. *Biochemistry* 1984, 23, 4232-6.

[42] Danesh, J., Lewington, S., Thompson, S. G., Lowe, G. D., Collins, R., Kostis, J. B., Wilson, A. C., Folsom, A. R., Wu, K., Benderly, M., Goldbourt, U., Willeit, J., Kiechl, S., Yarnell, J. W., Sweetnam, P. M., Elwood, P. C., Cushman, M., Psaty, B. M., Tracy, R. P., Tybjaerg-Hansen, A., Haverkate, F., de Maat, M. P., Fowkes, F. G., Lee, A. J., Smith, F. B., Salomaa, V., Harald, K., Rasi, R., Vahtera, E., Jousilahti, P., Pekkanen, J., D'Agostino, R., Kannel, W. B., Wilson, P. W., Tofler, G., Arocha-Piñango, C. L., Rodriguez-Larralde, A., Nagy, E., Mijares, M., Espinosa, R., Rodriquez-Roa, E., Ryder, E., Diez-Ewald, M. P., Campos, G., Fernandez, V., Torres, E., Marchioli, R., Valagussa, F., Rosengren, A., Wilhelmsen, L., Lappas, G., Eriksson, H., Cremer, P., Nagel, D., Curb, J. D., Rodriguez, B., Yano, K., Salonen, J. T., Nyyssönen, K., Tuomainen, T. P., Hedblad, B., Lind, P., Loewel, H., Koenig, W., Meade, T. W., Cooper, J. A., De Stavola, B., Knottenbelt, C., Miller, G. J., Bauer, K. A., Rosenberg, R. D., Sato, S., Kitamura, A., Naito, Y., Palosuo, T., Ducimetiere, P., Amouyel, P., Arveiler, D., Evans, A. E., Ferrieres, J., Juhan-Vague, I., Bingham, A., Schulte, H.,

Assmann, G., Cantin, B., Lamarche, B., Després, J. P., Dagenais, G. R., Tunstall-Pedoe, H., Woodward, M., Ben-Shlomo, Y., Davey Smith, G., Palmieri, V., Yeh, J. L., Rudnicka, A., Ridker, P., Rodeghiero, F., Tosetto, A., Shepherd, J., Ford, I., Robertson, M., Brunner, E., Shipley, M., Feskens, E. J., Kromhout, D., Dickinson, A., Ireland, B., Juzwishin, K., Kaptoge, S., Memon, A., Sarwar, N., Walker, M., Wheeler, J., White, I., Wood, A., Collaboration, F. S., Plasma fibrinogen level and the risk of major cardiovascular diseases and nonvascular mortality: an individual participant meta-analysis. *JAMA* 2005, 294, 1799-809.

[43] Ernst, E., Resch, K. L., Fibrinogen as a cardiovascular risk factor: a meta-analysis and review of the literature. *Ann. Intern. Med.* 1993, 118, 956-63.

[44] Wilhelmsen, L., Svärdsudd, K., Korsan-Bengtsen, K., Larsson, B., Welin, L., Tibblin, G., Fibrinogen as a risk factor for stroke and myocardial infarction. *N. Engl. J. Med.* 1984, 311, 501-5.

[45] Koster, T., Rosendaal, F. R., Reitsma, P. H., van der Velden, P. A., Briët, E., Vandenbroucke, J. P., Factor VII and fibrinogen levels as risk factors for venous thrombosis. A case-control study of plasma levels and DNA polymorphisms--the Leiden Thrombophilia Study (LETS). *Thromb. Haemost.* 1994, 71, 719-22.

[46] Uitte de Willige, S., de Visser, M. C., Houwing-Duistermaat, J. J., Rosendaal, F. R., Vos, H. L., Bertina, R. M., Genetic variation in the fibrinogen gamma gene increases the risk for deep venous thrombosis by reducing plasma fibrinogen gamma' levels. *Blood* 2005, 106, 4176-83.

[47] Souto, J. C., Almasy, L., Borrell, M., Garí, M., Martínez, E., Mateo, J., Stone, W. H., Blangero, J., Fontcuberta, J., Genetic determinants of hemostasis phenotypes in Spanish families. *Circulation* 2000, 101, 1546-51.

[48] De Lange, M., Snieder, H., Ariëns, R. A., Spector, T. D., Grant, P. J., The genetics of haemostasis: a twin study. *Lancet* 2001, 357, 101-5.

[49] Dehghan, A., Yang, Q., Peters, A., Basu, S., Bis, J. C., Rudnicka, A. R., Kavousi, M., Chen, M. H., Baumert, J., Lowe, G. D., McKnight, B., Tang, W., de Maat, M., Larson, M. G., Eyhermendy, S., McArdle, W. L., Lumley, T., Pankow, J. S., Hofman, A., Massaro, J. M., Rivadeneira, F., Kolz, M., Taylor, K. D., van Duijn, C. M., Kathiresan, S., Illig, T., Aulchenko, Y. S., Volcik, K. A., Johnson, A. D., Uitterlinden, A. G., Tofler, G. H., Gieger, C., Psaty, B. M., Couper, D. J., Boerwinkle, E., Koenig, W., O'Donnell, C. J., Witteman, J. C., Strachan, D. P., Smith, N. L., Folsom, A. R., Consortium, W. T. C. C., Association of novel genetic

Loci with circulating fibrinogen levels: a genome-wide association study in 6 population-based cohorts. *Circ. Cardiovasc. Genet.* 2009, 2, 125-33.

[50] Danik, J. S., Paré, G., Chasman, D. I., Zee, R. Y., Kwiatkowski, D. J., Parker, A., Miletich, J. P., Ridker, P. M., Novel loci, including those related to Crohn disease, psoriasis, and inflammation, identified in a genome-wide association study of fibrinogen in 17 686 women: the Women's Genome Health Study. *Circ. Cardiovasc. Genet.* 2009, 2, 134-41.

[51] Sabater-Lleal, M., Huang, J., Chasman, D., Naitza, S., Dehghan, A., Johnson, A. D., Teumer, A., Reiner, A. P., Folkersen, L., Basu, S., Rudnicka, A. R., Trompet, S., Mälarstig, A., Baumert, J., Bis, J. C., Guo, X., Hottenga, J. J., Shin, S. Y., Lopez, L. M., Lahti, J., Tanaka, T., Yanek, L. R., Oudot-Mellakh, T., Wilson, J. F., Navarro, P., Huffman, J. E., Zemunik, T., Redline, S., Mehra, R., Pulanic, D., Rudan, I., Wright, A. F., Kolcic, I., Polasek, O., Wild, S. H., Campbell, H., Curb, J. D., Wallace, R., Liu, S., Eaton, C. B., Becker, D. M., Becker, L. C., Bandinelli, S., Räikkönen, K., Widen, E., Palotie, A., Fornage, M., Green, D., Gross, M., Davies, G., Harris, S. E., Liewald, D. C., Starr, J. M., Williams, F. M., Grant, P. J., Spector, T. D., Strawbridge, R. J., Silveira, A., Sennblad, B., Rivadeneira, F., Uitterlinden, A. G., Franco, O. H., Hofman, A., van Dongen, J., Willemsen, G., Boomsma, D. I., Yao, J., Swords Jenny, N., Haritunians, T., McKnight, B., Lumley, T., Taylor, K. D., Rotter, J. I., Psaty, B. M., Peters, A., Gieger, C., Illig, T., Grotevendt, A., Homuth, G., Völzke, H., Kocher, T., Goel, A., Franzosi, M. G., Seedorf, U., Clarke, R., Steri, M., Tarasov, K. V., Sanna, S., Schlessinger, D., Stott, D. J., Sattar, N., Buckley, B. M., Rumley, A., Lowe, G. D., McArdle, W. L., Chen, M. H., Tofler, G. H., Song, J., Boerwinkle, E., Folsom, A. R., Rose, L. M., Franco-Cereceda, A., Teichert, M., Ikram, M. A., Mosley, T. H., Bevan, S., Dichgans, M., Rothwell, P. M., Sudlow, C. L., Hopewell, J. C., Chambers, J. C., Saleheen, D., Kooner, J. S., Danesh, J., Nelson, C. P., Erdmann, J., Reilly, M. P., Kathiresan, S., Schunkert, H., Morange, P. E., Ferrucci, L., Eriksson, J. G., Jacobs, D., Deary, I. J., Soranzo, N., Witteman, J. C., de Geus, E. J., Tracy, R. P., Hayward, C., Koenig, W., Cucca, F., Jukema, J. W., Eriksson, P., Seshadri, S., Markus, H. S., Watkins, H., Samani, N. J., Wallaschofski, H., Smith, N. L., Tregouet, D., Ridker, P. M., Tang, W., Strachan, D. P., Hamsten, A., O'Donnell, C. J., Consortium, V., Consortium, S., (WTCCC2), W. T. C. C. C.; Consortium, C. D.; Consortium, C., Multiethnic meta-analysis of genome-wide association

studies in >100 000 subjects identifies 23 fibrinogen-associated Loci but no strong evidence of a causal association between circulating fibrinogen and cardiovascular disease. *Circulation* 2013, 128, 1310-24.

[52] Stec, J. J., Silbershatz, H., Tofler, G. H., Matheney, T. H., Sutherland, P., Lipinska, I., Massaro, J. M., Wilson, P. F., Muller, J. E., D'Agostino, R. B., Association of fibrinogen with cardiovascular risk factors and cardiovascular disease in the Framingham Offspring Population. *Circulation* 2000, 102, 1634-8.

[53] Kim, P. Y., Stewart, R. J., Lipson, S. M., Nesheim, M. E., The relative kinetics of clotting and lysis provide a biochemical rationale for the correlation between elevated fibrinogen and cardiovascular disease. *J. Thromb. Haemost.* 2007, 5, 1250-6.

[54] Falls, L. A., Farrell, D. H., Resistance of gammaA/gamma' fibrin clots to fibrinolysis. *J. Biol. Chem.* 1997, 272, 14251-6.

[55] Grünbacher, G., Weger, W., Marx-Neuhold, E., Pilger, E., Köppel, H., Wascher, T., März, W., Renner, W., The fibrinogen gamma (FGG) 10034C>T polymorphism is associated with venous thrombosis. *Thromb. Res.* 2007, 121, 33-6.

[56] Lovely, R. S., Yang, Q., Massaro, J. M., Wang, J., D'Agostino, R. B., O'Donnell, C. J., Shannon, J., Farrell, D. H., Assessment of genetic determinants of the association of γ' fibrinogen in relation to cardiovascular disease. *Arterioscler. Thromb. Vasc. Biol.* 2011, 31, 2345-52.

[57] Standeven, K. F., Grant, P. J., Carter, A. M., Scheiner, T., Weisel, J. W., Ariëns, R. A., Functional analysis of the fibrinogen Aalpha Thr312Ala polymorphism: effects on fibrin structure and function. *Circulation* 2003, 107, 2326-30.

[58] Mosesson, M. W., Update on antithrombin I (fibrin). *Thromb. Haemost.* 2007, 98, 105-8.

[59] Drouet, L., Paolucci, F., Pasqualini, N., Laprade, M., Ripoll, L., Mazoyer, E., Bal dit Sollier, C., Vanhove, N., Plasma gamma'/gamma fibrinogen ratio, a marker of arterial thrombotic activity: a new potential cardiovascular risk factor? *Blood Coagul. Fibrinolysis* 1999, 10 Suppl. 1, S35-9.

[60] Uitte de Willige, S., Standeven, K. F., Philippou, H., Ariëns, R. A., The pleiotropic role of the fibrinogen gamma' chain in hemostasis. *Blood* 2009, 114, 3994-4001.

[61] Petrera, N. S., Stafford, A. R., Leslie, B. A., Kretz, C. A., Fredenburgh, J. C., Weitz, J. I., Long range communication between exosites 1 and 2 modulates thrombin function. *J. Biol. Chem.* 2009, 284, 25620-9.

[62] Lovely, R. S., Rein, C. M., White, T. C., Jouihan, S. A., Boshkov, L. K., Bakke, A. C., McCarty, O. J., Farrell, D. H., gammaA/gamma' fibrinogen inhibits thrombin-induced platelet aggregation. *Thromb. Haemost.* 2008, 100, 837-46.

[63] Lancellotti, S., Rutella, S., De Filippis, V., Pozzi, N., Rocca, B., De Cristofaro, R., Fibrinogen-elongated gamma chain inhibits thrombin-induced platelet response, hindering the interaction with different receptors. *J. Biol. Chem.* 2008, 283, 30193-204.

[64] Mosesson, M. W., Cooley, B. C., Hernandez, I., Diorio, J. P., Weiler, H., Thrombosis risk modification in transgenic mice containing the human fibrinogen thrombin-binding gamma' chain sequence. *J. Thromb. Haemost.* 2009, 7, 102-10.

[65] Cheung, E. Y., Vos, H. L., Kruip, M. J., den Hertog, H. M., Jukema, J. W., de Maat, M. P., Elevated fibrinogen gamma' ratio is associated with cardiovascular diseases and acute phase reaction but not with clinical outcome. *Blood* 2009, 114, 4603-4; author reply 4604-5.

[66] Weiler, H., Mouse models of thrombosis: thrombomodulin. *Thromb. Haemost.* 2004, 92, 467-77.

[67] De Candia, E., Hall, S. W., Rutella, S., Landolfi, R., Andrews, R. K., De Cristofaro, R., Binding of thrombin to glycoprotein Ib accelerates the hydrolysis of Par-1 on intact platelets. *J. Biol. Chem.* 2001, 276, 4692-8.

[68] Fredenburgh, J. C., Stafford, A. R., Leslie, B. A., Weitz, J. I., Bivalent binding to gammaA/gamma'-fibrin engages both exosites of thrombin and protects it from inhibition by the antithrombin-heparin complex. *J. Biol. Chem.* 2008, 283, 2470-7.

[69] Olds, R. J., Lane, D. A., Mille, B., Chowdhury, V., Thein, S. L., Antithrombin: the principal inhibitor of thrombin. *Semin. Thromb. Hemost.* 1994, 20, 353-72.

[70] Bedsted, T., Swanson, R., Chuang, Y. J., Bock, P. E., Björk, I., Olson, S. T., Heparin and calcium ions dramatically enhance antithrombin reactivity with factor IXa by generating new interaction exosites. *Biochemistry* 2003, 42, 8143-52.

[71] Rau, J., Beaulieu, L., Huntington, J., Church, F., Serpins in thrombosis, hemostasis and fibrinolysis. *J. Thromb. Haemost.* 2007, 5 (Suppl. 1), 102-105.

[72] Bucciarelli, P., Passamonti, S. M., Biguzzi, E., Gianniello, F., Franchi, F., Mannucci, P. M., Martinelli, I., Low borderline plasma levels of antithrombin, protein C and protein S are risk factors for venous thromboembolism. *J. Thromb. Haemost.* 2012, 10, 1783-91.

[73] Egeberg, O., Inherited antithrombin deficiency causing thrombophilia. *Thromb. Diath. Haemorrh.* 1965, 13, 516-530.

[74] Lijfering, W. M., Brouwer, J. L., Veeger, N. J., Bank, I., Coppens, M., Middeldorp, S., Hamulyák, K., Prins, M. H., Büller, H. R., van der Meer, J., Selective testing for thrombophilia in patients with first venous thrombosis: results from a retrospective family cohort study on absolute thrombotic risk for currently known thrombophilic defects in 2479 relatives. *Blood* 2009, 113, 5314-22.

[75] Ishiguro, K., Kojima, T., Kadomatsu, K., Nakayama, Y., Takagi, A., Suzuki, M., Takeda, N., Ito, M., Yamamoto, K., Matsushita, T., Kusugami, K., Muramatsu, T., Saito, H., Complete antithrombin deficiency in mice results in embryonic lethality. *J. Clin. Invest.* 2000, 106, 873-8.

[76] Lane, D. *Antithrombin mutation database*. (accessed 21/11/2013).

[77] Cooper, D., Krawczak, M. *Human gene mutation database*. (accessed 21/11/2013).

[78] Luxembourg, B., Delev, D., Geisen, C., Spannagl, M., Krause, M., Miesbach, W., Heller, C., Bergmann, F., Schmeink, U., Grossmann, R., Lindhoff-Last, E., Seifried, E., Oldenburg, J., Pavlova, A., Molecular basis of antithrombin deficiency. *Thromb. Haemost.* 2011, 105, 635-46.

[79] Antón, A. I., Teruel, R., Corral, J., Miñano, A., Martínez-Martínez, I., Ordóñez, A., Vicente, V., Sánchez-Vega, B., Functional consequences of the prothrombotic SERPINC1 rs2227589 polymorphism on antithrombin levels. *Haematologica* 2009, 94, 589-92.

[80] Oudot-Mellakh, T., Cohen, W., Germain, M., Saut, N., Kallel, C., Zelenika, D., Lathrop, M., Trégouët, D. A., Morange, P. E., Genome wide association study for plasma levels of natural anticoagulant inhibitors and protein C anticoagulant pathway: the MARTHA project. *Br. J. Haematol.* 2012, 157, 230-9.

[81] Lane, D. A., Bayston, T., Olds, R. J., Fitches, A. C., Cooper, D. N., Millar, D. S., Jochmans, K., Perry, D. J., Okajima, K., Thein, S. L., Emmerich, J., Antithrombin mutation database: 2nd (1997) update. For the Plasma Coagulation Inhibitors Subcommittee of the Scientific and Standardization Committee of the International Society on Thrombosis and Haemostasis. *Thromb. Haemost.* 1997, 77, 197-211.

[82] Martínez-Martínez, I., Navarro-Fernández, J., Østergaard, A., Gutiérrez-Gallego, R., Padilla, J., Bohdan, N., Miñano, A., Pascual, C., Martínez, C., de la Morena-Barrio, M. E., Aguila, S., Pedersen, S., Kristensen, S. R., Vicente, V., Corral, J., Amelioration of the severity of heparin-binding antithrombin mutations by posttranslational mosaicism. *Blood* 2012, 120, 900-4.

[83] Corral, J., Hernandez-Espinosa, D., Soria, J. M., Gonzalez-Conejero, R., Ordonez, A., Gonzalez-Porras, J. R., Perez-Ceballos, E., Lecumberri, R., Sanchez, I., Roldan, V., Mateo, J., Minano, A., Gonzalez, M., Alberca, I., Fontcuberta, J., Vicente, V., Antithrombin Cambridge II (A384S): an underestimated genetic risk factor for venous thrombosis. *Blood* 2007, 109, 4258-63.

[84] Mushunje, A., Zhou, A., Carrell, R. W., Huntington, J. A., Heparin-induced substrate behavior of antithrombin Cambridge II. *Blood* 2003, 102, 4028-34.

[85] Sanchez, C., Alessi, M. C., Saut, N., Aillaud, M. F., Morange, P. E., Relation between the antithrombin Cambridge II mutation, the risk of venous thrombosis, and the endogenous thrombin generation. *J. Thromb. Haemost.* 2008, 6, 1975-7.

[86] Roldán, V., Ordoñez, A., Marín, F., Zorio, E., Soria, J. M., Miñano, A., España, F., González-Conejero, R., Pineda, J., Estellés, A., Fontcuberta, J., Vicente, V., Corral, J., Antithrombin Cambridge II (A384S) supports a role for antithrombin deficiency in arterial thrombosis. *Thromb. Haemost.* 2009, 101, 483-6.

[87] Vossen, C. Y., Conard, J., Fontcuberta, J., Makris, M., Van der Meer, F. J., Pabinger, I., Palareti, G., Preston, F. E., Scharrer, I., Souto, J. C., Svensson, P., Walker, I. D., Rosendaal, F. R., Risk of a first venous thrombotic event in carriers of a familial thrombophilic defect. The European Prospective Cohort on Thrombophilia (EPCOT). *J. Thromb. Haemost.* 2005, 3, 459-64.

[88] Rossi, E., Ciminello, A., Za, T., Betti, S., Leone, G., De Stefano, V., In families with inherited thrombophilia the risk of venous thromboembolism is dependent on the clinical phenotype of the proband. *Thromb. Haemost.* 2011, 106, 646-54.

[89] Holzhauer, S., Goldenberg, N. A., Junker, R., Heller, C., Stoll, M., Manner, D., Mesters, R., Krümpel, A., Stach, M., Nowak-Göttl, U., Inherited thrombophilia in children with venous thromboembolism and the familial risk of thromboembolism: an observational study. *Blood* 2012, 120, 1510-5.

[90] Finazzi, G., Caccia, R., Barbui, T., Different prevalence of thromboembolism in the subtypes of congenital antithrombin III deficiency: review of 404 cases. *Thromb. Haemost.* 1987, 58, 1094.

[91] Luxembourg, B., Pavlova, A., Geisen, C., Spannagl, M., Bergmann, F., Krause, M., Alesci, S., Seifried, E., Lindhoff-Last, E., Impact of the type of SERPINC1 mutation and subtype of antithrombin deficiency on the thrombotic phenotype in hereditary antithrombin deficiency. *Thromb. Haemost.* 2013, 111.

[92] Estellés, A., Garcia-Plaza, I., Dasí, A., Aznar, J., Duart, M., Sanz, G., Pérez-Requejo, J. L., España, F., Jimenez, C., Abeledo, G., Severe inherited "homozygous" protein C deficiency in a newborn infant. *Thromb. Haemost.* 1984, 52, 53-6.

[93] Stearns-Kurosawa, D. J., Kurosawa, S., Mollica, J. S., Ferrell, G. L., Esmon, C. T., The endothelial cell protein C receptor augments protein C activation by the thrombin-thrombomodulin complex. *Proc. Natl. Acad. Sci. US* 1996, 93, 10212-6.

[94] Walker, F. J., Regulation of activated protein C by protein S. The role of phospholipid in factor Va inactivation. *J. Biol. Chem.* 1981, 256, 11128-31.

[95] Fulcher, C. A., Gardiner, J. E., Griffin, J. H., Zimmerman, T. S., Proteolytic inactivation of human factor VIII procoagulant protein by activated human protein C and its analogy with factor V. *Blood* 1984, 63, 486-9.

[96] Danese, S., Vetrano, S., Zhang, L., Poplis, V. A., Castellino, F. J., The protein C pathway in tissue inflammation and injury: pathogenic role and therapeutic implications. *Blood* 2010, 115, 1121-30.

[97] Weiler, H., Multiple receptor-mediated functions of activated protein C. *Hamostaseologie* 2011, 31, 185-95.

[98] Seligsohn, U., Berger, A., Abend, M., Rubin, L., Attias, D., Zivelin, A., Rapaport, S. I., Homozygous protein C deficiency manifested by massive venous thrombosis in the newborn. *N. Engl. J. Med.* 1984, 310, 559-62.

[99] Folsom, A. R., Aleksic, N., Wang, L., Cushman, M., Wu, K. K., White, R. H., Protein C, antithrombin, and venous thromboembolism incidence: a prospective population-based study. *Arterioscler. Thromb. Vasc. Biol.* 2002, 22, 1018-22.

[100] España, F., Vayá, A., Mira, Y., Medina, P., Estellés, A., Villa, P., Falcó, C., Aznar, J., Low level of circulating activated protein C is a risk factor for venous thromboembolism. *Thromb. Haemost.* 2001, 86, 1368-73.

[101] Spek, C. A., Koster, T., Rosendaal, F. R., Bertina, R. M., Reitsma, P. H., Genotypic variation in the promoter region of the protein C gene is associated with plasma protein C levels and thrombotic risk. *Arterioscler. Thromb. Vasc. Biol.* 1995, 15, 214-8.

[102] Aiach, M., Nicaud, V., Alhenc-Gelas, M., Gandrille, S., Arnaud, E., Amiral, J., Guize, L., Fiessinger, J. N., Emmerich, J., Complex association of protein C gene promoter polymorphism with circulating protein C levels and thrombotic risk. *Arterioscler. Thromb. Vasc. Biol.* 1999, 19, 1573-6.

[103] Reiner, A. P., Carty, C. L., Jenny, N. S., Nievergelt, C., Cushman, M., Stearns-Kurosawa, D. J., Kurosawa, S., Kuller, L. H., Lange, L. A., PROC, PROCR and PROS1 polymorphisms, plasma anticoagulant phenotypes, and risk of cardiovascular disease and mortality in older adults: the Cardiovascular Health Study. *J. Thromb. Haemost.* 2008, 6, 1625-32.

[104] Pintao, M. C., Roshani, S., de Visser, M. C., Tieken, C., Tanck, M. W., Wichers, I. M., Meijers, J. C., Rosendaal, F. R., Middeldorp, S., Reitsma, P. H., High levels of protein C are determined by PROCR haplotype 3. *J. Thromb. Haemost.* 2011, 9, 969-76.

[105] Tang, W., Basu, S., Kong, X., Pankow, J. S., Aleksic, N., Tan, A., Cushman, M., Boerwinkle, E., Folsom, A. R., Genome-wide association study identifies novel loci for plasma levels of protein C: the ARIC study. *Blood* 2010, 116, 5032-6.

[106] Reitsma, P. H., Bernardi, F., Doig, R. G., Gandrille, S., Greengard, J. S., Ireland, H., Krawczak, M., Lind, B., Long, G. L., Poort, S. R., Protein C deficiency: a database of mutations, 1995 update. On behalf of the Subcommittee on Plasma Coagulation Inhibitors of the Scientific and Standardization Committee of the ISTH. *Thromb. Haemost.* 1995, 73, 876-89.

[107] Gandrille, S., Aiach, M., Identification of mutations in 90 of 121 consecutive symptomatic French patients with a type I protein C deficiency. The French INSERM Network on Molecular Abnormalities Responsible for Protein C and Protein S deficiencies. *Blood* 1995, 86, 2598-605.

[108] Alhenc-Gelas, M., Gandrille, S., Aubry, M. L., Aiach, M., Thirty-three novel mutations in the protein C gene. French INSERM network on molecular abnormalities responsible for protein C and protein S. *Thromb. Haemost.* 2000, 83, 86-92.

[109] Gandrille, S., Alhenc-Gelas, M., Gaussem, P., Aillaud, M. F., Dupuy, E., Juhan-Vague, I., Aiach, M., Five novel mutations located in exons III and IX of the protein C gene in patients presenting with defective protein C anticoagulant activity. *Blood* 1993, 82, 159-68.

[110] Fisher, C. L., Greengard, J. S., Griffin, J. H., Models of the serine protease domain of the human antithrombotic plasma factor activated protein C and its zymogen. *Protein Sci.* 1994, 3, 588-99.

[111] Vincenot, A., Gaussem, P., Pittet, J. L., Debost, S., Aiach, M., Amino acids 225-235** of the protein C serine-protease domain are important for the interaction with the thrombin-thrombomodulin complex. *FEBS Lett.* 1995, 367, 153-7.

[112] Walker, F. J., Protein S and the regulation of activated protein C. *Semin. Thromb. Hemost.* 1984, 10, 131-8.

[113] Esmon, C. T., Vigano-D'Angelo, S., D'Angelo, A., Comp, P. C., Anticoagulation proteins C and S. *Adv. Exp. Med. Biol.* 1987, 214, 47-54.

[114] Esmon, N. L., D'Angelo, A., Vigano-D'Angelo, S., Esmon, C. T., Comp, P. C., Analysis of protein C and protein S in disease states. *Dev. Biol. Stand.* 1987, 67, 75-82.

[115] Hackeng, T. M., Seré, K. M., Tans, G., Rosing, J., Protein S stimulates inhibition of the tissue factor pathway by tissue factor pathway inhibitor. *Proc. Natl. Acad. Sci. US* 2006, 103, 3106-11.

[116] Dahlbäck, B., The tale of protein S and C4b-binding protein, a story of affection. *Thromb. Haemost.* 2007, 98, 90-6.

[117] Lane, D. A., Mannucci, P. M., Bauer, K. A., Bertina, R. M., Bochkov, N. P., Boulyjenkov, V., Chandy, M., Dahlbäck, B., Ginter, E. K., Miletich, J. P., Rosendaal, F. R., Seligsohn, U., Inherited thrombophilia: Part 2. *Thromb. Haemost.* 1996, 76, 824-34.

[118] Faioni, E. M., Valsecchi, C., Palla, A., Taioli, E., Razzari, C., Mannucci, P. M., Free protein S deficiency is a risk factor for venous thrombosis. *Thromb. Haemost.* 1997, 78, 1343-6.

[119] Martinelli, I., Mannucci, P. M., De Stefano, V., Taioli, E., Rossi, V., Crosti, F., Paciaroni, K., Leone, G., Faioni, E. M., Different risks of thrombosis in four coagulation defects associated with inherited thrombophilia: a study of 150 families. *Blood* 1998, 92, 2353-8.

[120] Makris, M., Leach, M., Beauchamp, N. J., Daly, M. E., Cooper, P. C., Hampton, K. K., Bayliss, P., Peake, I. R., Miller, G. J., Preston, F. E., Genetic analysis, phenotypic diagnosis, and risk of venous thrombosis in

families with inherited deficiencies of protein S. *Blood* 2000, 95, 1935-41.

[121] Beauchamp, N. J., Dykes, A. C., Parikh, N., Campbell Tait, R., Daly, M. E., The prevalence of, and molecular defects underlying, inherited protein S deficiency in the general population. *Br. J. Haematol.* 2004, 125, 647-54.

[122] Koster, T., Rosendaal, F. R., Briët, E., van der Meer, F. J., Colly, L. P., Trienekens, P. H., Poort, S. R., Reitsma, P. H., Vandenbroucke, J. P., Protein C deficiency in a controlled series of unselected outpatients: an infrequent but clear risk factor for venous thrombosis (Leiden Thrombophilia Study). *Blood* 1995, 85, 2756-61.

[123] Liberti, G., Bertina, R. M., Rosendaal, F. R., Hormonal state rather than age influences cut-off values of protein S: reevaluation of the thrombotic risk associated with protein S deficiency. *Thromb. Haemost.* 1999, 82, 1093-6.

[124] Boyer-Neumann, C., Bertina, R. M., Tripodi, A., D'Angelo, A., Wolf, M., Vigano D'Angelo, S., Mannucci, P. M., Meyer, D., Larrieu, M. J., Comparison of functional assays for protein S: European collaborative study of patients with congenital and acquired deficiency. *Thromb. Haemost.* 1993, 70, 946-50.

[125] Fernández, J. A., Estellés, A., Gilabert, J., España, F., Aznar, J., Functional and immunologic protein S in normal pregnant women and in full-term newborns. *Thromb. Haemost.* 1989, 61, 474-8.

[126] García de Frutos, P., Alim, R. I., Härdig, Y., Zöller, B., Dahlbäck, B., Differential regulation of alpha and beta chains of C4b-binding protein during acute-phase response resulting in stable plasma levels of free anticoagulant protein S. *Blood* 1994, 84, 815-22.

[127] Henkens, C. M., Bom, V. J., Van der Schaaf, W., Pelsma, P. M., Sibinga, C. T., de Kam, P. J., van der Meer, J., Plasma levels of protein S, protein C, and factor X: effects of sex, hormonal state and age. *Thromb. Haemost.* 1995, 74, 1271-5.

[128] D'Angelo, A., Viganò D'Angelo, S., Protein S deficiency. *Haematologica* 2008, 93, 498-501.

[129] Comp, P. C., Nixon, R. R., Cooper, M. R., Esmon, C. T., Familial protein S deficiency is associated with recurrent thrombosis. *J. Clin. Invest.* 1984, 74, 2082-8.

[130] Comp, P. C., Esmon, C. T., Recurrent venous thromboembolism in patients with a partial deficiency of protein S. *N. Engl. J. Med.* 1984, 311, 1525-8.

[131] Gandrille, S., Borgel, D., Sala, N., Espinosa-Parrilla, Y., Simmonds, R., Rezende, S., Lind, B., Mannhalter, C., Pabinger, I., Reitsma, P. H., Formstone, C., Cooper, D. N., Saito, H., Suzuki, K., Bernardi, F., Aiach, M., Haemostasis, P. C. I. S. o. t. S. a. S. C. o. t. I. S. o. T. a., Protein S deficiency: a database of mutations--summary of the first update. *Thromb. Haemost.* 2000, 84, 918.

[132] García de Frutos, P., Fuentes-Prior, P., Hurtado, B., Sala, N., Molecular basis of protein S deficiency. *Thromb. Haemost.* 2007, 98, 543-56.

[133] Castoldi, E., Maurissen, L. F., Tormene, D., Spiezia, L., Gavasso, S., Radu, C., Hackeng, T. M., Rosing, J., Simioni, P., Similar hypercoagulable state and thrombosis risk in type I and type III protein S-deficient individuals from mixed type I/III families. *Haematologica* 2010.

[134] Johansson, A. M., Hillarp, A., Säll, T., Zöller, B., Dahlbäck, B., Halldén, C., Large deletions of the PROS1 gene in a large fraction of mutation-negative patients with protein S deficiency. *Thromb. Haemost.* 2005, 94, 951-7.

[135] Pintao, M. C., Garcia, A. A., Borgel, D., Alhenc-Gelas, M., Spek, C. A., de Visser, M. C., Gandrille, S., Reitsma, P. H., Gross deletions/ duplications in PROS1 are relatively common in point mutation-negative hereditary protein S deficiency. *Hum. Genet.* 2009, 126, 449-56.

[136] Bertina, R. M., Ploos van Amstel, H. K., van Wijngaarden, A., Coenen, J., Leemhuis, M. P., Deutz-Terlouw, P. P., van der Linden, I. K., Reitsma, P. H., Heerlen polymorphism of protein S, an immunologic polymorphism due to dimorphism of residue 460. *Blood* 1990, 76, 538-48.

[137] Duchemin, J., Gandrille, S., Borgel, D., Feurgard, P., Alhenc-Gelas, M., Matheron, C., Dreyfus, M., Dupuy, E., Juhan-Vague, I., Aiach, M., The Ser 460 to Pro substitution of the protein S alpha (PROS1) gene is a frequent mutation associated with free protein S (type IIa) deficiency. *Blood* 1995, 86, 3436-43.

[138] Athanasiadis, G., Buil, A., Souto, J. C., Borrell, M., López, S.; Martinez-Perez, A., Lathrop, M., Fontcuberta, J., Almasy, L., Soria, J. M., A genome-wide association study of the Protein C anticoagulant pathway. *PLoS One* 2011, 6, e29168.

[139] Koster, T., Blann, A. D., Briët, E., Vandenbroucke, J. P., Rosendaal, F. R., Role of clotting factor VIII in effect of von Willebrand factor on occurrence of deep-vein thrombosis. *Lancet* 1995, 345, 152-5.

[140] Franchini, M., Capra, F., Targher, G., Montagnana, M., Lippi, G., Relationship between ABO blood group and von Willebrand factor levels: from biology to clinical implications. *Thromb. J.* 2007, 5, 14.
[141] Gill, J. C., Endres-Brooks, J., Bauer, P. J., Marks, W. J., Montgomery, R. R., The effect of ABO blood group on the diagnosis of von Willebrand disease. *Blood* 1987, 69, 1691-5.
[142] Franchini, M., Makris, M., Non-O blood group: an important genetic risk factor for venous thromboembolism. *Blood Transfus.* 2013, 11, 164-5.
[143] Wautrecht, J. C., Galle, C., Motte, S., Dereume, J. P., Dramaix, M., The role of ABO blood groups in the incidence of deep vein thrombosis. *Thromb. Haemost.* 1998, 79, 688-9.
[144] Spiezia, L., Campello, E., Bon, M., Tison, T., Milan, M., Simioni, P., Prandoni, P., ABO blood groups and the risk of venous thrombosis in patients with inherited thrombophilia. *Blood Transfus.* 2013, 11, 250-3.
[145] Tirado, I., Mateo, J., Soria, J. M., Oliver, A., Martínez-Sánchez, E., Vallvé, C., Borrell, M., Urrutia, T., Fontcuberta, J., The ABO blood group genotype and factor VIII levels as independent risk factors for venous thromboembolism. *Thromb. Haemost.* 2005, 93, 468-74.
[146] Ohira, T., Cushman, M., Tsai, M. Y., Zhang, Y., Heckbert, S. R., Zakai, N. A., Rosamond, W. D., Folsom, A. R., ABO blood group, other risk factors and incidence of venous thromboembolism: the Longitudinal Investigation of Thromboembolism Etiology (LITE). *J. Thromb. Haemost.* 2007, 5, 1455-61.
[147] Wu, O., Bayoumi, N., Vickers, M. A., Clark, P., ABO(H) blood groups and vascular disease: a systematic review and meta-analysis. *J. Thromb. Haemost.* 2008, 6, 62-9.
[148] Jick, H., Slone, D., Westerholm, B., Inman, W. H., Vessey, M. P., Shapiro, S., Lewis, G. P., Worcester, J., Venous thromboembolic disease and ABO blood type. A cooperative study. *Lancet* 1969, 1, 539-42.
[149] Heit, J. A., Armasu, S. M., Asmann, Y. W., Cunningham, J. M., Matsumoto, M. E., Petterson, T. M., De Andrade, M., A genome-wide association study of venous thromboembolism identifies risk variants in chromosomes 1q24.2 and 9q. *J. Thromb. Haemost.* 2012, 10, 1521-31.
[150] Germain, M., Saut, N., Greliche, N., Dina, C., Lambert, J. C., Perret, C., Cohen, W., Oudot-Mellakh, T., Antoni, G., Alessi, M. C., Zelenika, D., Cambien, F., Tiret, L., Bertrand, M., Dupuy, A. M., Letenneur, L., Lathrop, M., Emmerich, J., Amouyel, P., Trégouët, D. A., Morange, P.

E., Genetics of venous thrombosis: insights from a new genome wide association study. *PLoS One* 2011, 6, e25581.

[151] Heit, J. A., Cunningham, J. M., Petterson, T. M., Armasu, S. M., Rider, D. N., De Andrade, M., Genetic variation within the anticoagulant, procoagulant, fibrinolytic and innate immunity pathways as risk factors for venous thromboembolism. *J. Thromb. Haemost.* 2011, 9, 1133-42.

[152] Jenkins, P. V., O'Donnell, J. S., ABO blood group determines plasma von Willebrand factor levels: a biologic function after all? *Transfusion* 2006, 46, 1836-44.

[153] McGrath, R. T., McKinnon, T. A., Byrne, B., O'Kennedy, R., Terraube, V., McRae, E., Preston, R. J., Laffan, M. A., O'Donnell, J. S., Expression of terminal alpha2-6-linked sialic acid on von Willebrand factor specifically enhances proteolysis by ADAMTS13. *Blood* 2010, 115, 2666-73.

[154] Cohen, W., Castelli, C., Alessi, M. C., Aillaud, M. F., Bouvet, S., Saut, N., Brunet, D., Barthet, M. C., Tregouet, D. A., Lavigne, G., Morange, P. E., ABO blood group and von Willebrand factor levels partially explained the incomplete penetrance of congenital thrombophilia. *Arterioscler. Thromb. Vasc. Biol.* 2012, 32, 2021-8.

[155] Kiechl, S., Paré, G., Barbalic, M., Qi, L., Dupuis, J., Dehghan, A., Bis, J. C., Laxton, R. C., Xiao, Q., Bonora, E., Willeit, J., Xu, Q., Witteman, J. C., Chasman, D., Tracy, R. P., Ballantyne, C. M., Ridker, P. M., Benjamin, E. J., Ye, S., Association of variation at the ABO locus with circulating levels of soluble intercellular adhesion molecule-1, soluble P-selectin, and soluble E-selectin: a meta-analysis. *Circ. Cardiovasc. Genet.* 2011, 4, 681-6.

[156] Smith, N. L., Rice, K. M., Bovill, E. G., Cushman, M., Bis, J. C., McKnight, B., Lumley, T., Glazer, N. L., van Hylckama Vlieg, A., Tang, W., Dehghan, A., Strachan, D. P., O'Donnell, C. J., Rotter, J. I., Heckbert, S. R., Psaty, B. M., Rosendaal, F. R., Genetic variation associated with plasma von Willebrand factor levels and the risk of incident venous thrombosis. *Blood* 2011, 117, 6007-11.

[157] Smith, N. L., Chen, M. H., Dehghan, A., Strachan, D. P., Basu, S., Soranzo, N., Hayward, C., Rudan, I., Sabater-Lleal, M., Bis, J. C., de Maat, M. P., Rumley, A., Kong, X., Yang, Q., Williams, F. M., Vitart, V., Campbell, H., Mälarstig, A., Wiggins, K. L., Van Duijn, C. M., McArdle, W. L., Pankow, J. S., Johnson, A. D., Silveira, A., McKnight, B., Uitterlinden, A. G., Aleksic, N., Meigs, J. B., Peters, A., Koenig, W., Cushman, M., Kathiresan, S., Rotter, J. I., Bovill, E. G., Hofman, A.,

Boerwinkle, E., Tofler, G. H., Peden, J. F., Psaty, B. M., Leebeek, F., Folsom, A. R., Larson, M. G., Spector, T. D., Wright, A. F., Wilson, J. F., Hamsten, A., Lumley, T., Witteman, J. C., Tang, W., O'Donnell, C. J., Consortium, W. T. C. C., Novel associations of multiple genetic loci with plasma levels of factor VII, factor VIII, and von Willebrand factor: The CHARGE (Cohorts for Heart and Aging Research in Genome Epidemiology) Consortium. *Circulation* 2010, 121, 1382-92.

[158] Antoni, G., Morange, P. E., Luo, Y., Saut, N., Burgos, G., Heath, S., Germain, M., Biron-Andreani, C., Schved, J. F., Pernod, G., Galan, P., Zelenika, D., Alessi, M. C., Drouet, L., Visvikis-Siest, S., Wells, P. S., Lathrop, M., Emmerich, J., Tregouet, D. A., Gagnon, F., A multi-stage multi-design strategy provides strong evidence that the BAI3 locus is associated with early-onset venous thromboembolism. *J. Thromb. Haemost.* 2010, 8, 2671-9.

[159] Van Loon, J. E., Sanders, Y. V., de Wee, E. M., Kruip, M. J., de Maat, M. P., Leebeek, F. W., Effect of genetic variation in STXBP5 and STX2 on von Willebrand factor and bleeding phenotype in type 1 von Willebrand disease patients. *PLoS One* 2012, 7, e40624.

[160] Meijers, J. C., Tekelenburg, W. L., Bouma, B. N., Bertina, R. M., Rosendaal, F. R., High levels of coagulation factor XI as a risk factor for venous thrombosis. *N. Engl. J. Med.* 2000, 342, 696-701.

[161] Gailani, D., Broze, G. J., Factor XI activation in a revised model of blood coagulation. *Science* 1991, 253, 909-12.

[162] Naito, K., Fujikawa, K., Activation of human blood coagulation factor XI independent of factor XII. Factor XI is activated by thrombin and factor XIa in the presence of negatively charged surfaces. *J. Biol. Chem.* 1991, 266, 7353-8.

[163] Amundadottir, L., Kraft, P., Stolzenberg-Solomon, R. Z., Fuchs, C. S., Petersen, G. M., Arslan, A. A., Bueno-de-Mesquita, H. B., Gross, M., Helzlsouer, K., Jacobs, E. J., LaCroix, A., Zheng, W., Albanes, D., Bamlet, W., Berg, C. D., Berrino, F., Bingham, S., Buring, J. E., Bracci, P. M., Canzian, F., Clavel-Chapelon, F., Clipp, S., Cotterchio, M., de Andrade, M., Duell, E. J., Fox, J. W., Gallinger, S., Gaziano, J. M., Giovannucci, E. L., Goggins, M., González, C. A., Hallmans, G., Hankinson, S. E., Hassan, M., Holly, E. A., Hunter, D. J., Hutchinson, A., Jackson, R., Jacobs, K. B., Jenab, M., Kaaks, R., Klein, A. P., Kooperberg, C., Kurtz, R. C., Li, D., Lynch, S. M., Mandelson, M., McWilliams, R. R., Mendelsohn, J. B., Michaud, D. S., Olson, S. H., Overvad, K., Patel, A. V., Peeters, P. H., Rajkovic, A., Riboli, E., Risch,

H. A., Shu, X. O., Thomas, G., Tobias, G. S., Trichopoulos, D., Van Den Eeden, S. K., Virtamo, J., Wactawski-Wende, J., Wolpin, B. M., Yu, H., Yu, K., Zeleniuch-Jacquotte, A., Chanock, S. J., Hartge, P., Hoover, R. N., Genome-wide association study identifies variants in the ABO locus associated with susceptibility to pancreatic cancer. *Nat. Genet.* 2009, 41, 986-90.

[164] Austin, H., De Staercke, C., Lally, C., Bezemer, I. D., Rosendaal, F. R., Hooper, W. C., New gene variants associated with venous thrombosis: a replication study in White and Black Americans. *J. Thromb. Haemost.* 2011, 9, 489-95.

[165] Snoep, J. D., Gaussem, P., Eikenboom, J. C., Emmerich, J., Zwaginga, J. J., Holmes, C. E., Vos, H. L., de Groot, P. G., Herrington, D. M., Bray, P. F., Rosendaal, F. R., van der Bom, J. G., The minor allele of GP6 T13254C is associated with decreased platelet activation and a reduced risk of recurrent cardiovascular events and mortality: results from the SMILE-Platelets project. *J. Thromb. Haemost.* 2010, 8, 2377-84.

[166] Vanschoonbeek, K., Feijge, M. A., Van Kampen, R. J., Kenis, H., Hemker, H. C., Giesen, P. L., Heemskerk, J. W., Initiating and potentiating role of platelets in tissue factor-induced thrombin generation in the presence of plasma: subject-dependent variation in thrombogram characteristics. *J. Thromb. Haemost.* 2004, 2, 476-84.

[167] Kotuličová, D., Chudý, P., Škereňová, M., Ivanková, J., Dobrotová, M., Kubisz, P., Variability of GP6 gene in patients with sticky platelet syndrome and deep venous thrombosis and/or pulmonary embolism. *Blood Coagul. Fibrinolysis* 2012, 23, 543-7.

[168] Fukudome, K., Esmon, C. T., Identification, cloning, and regulation of a novel endothelial cell protein C/activated protein C receptor. *J. Biol. Chem.* 1994, 269, 26486-91.

[169] Laszik, Z. G., Zhou, X. J., Ferrell, G. L., Silva, F. G., Esmon, C. T., Down-regulation of endothelial expression of endothelial cell protein C receptor and thrombomodulin in coronary atherosclerosis. *Am. J. Pathol.* 2001, 159, 797-802.

[170] Galligan, L., Livingstone, W., Volkov, Y., Hokamp, K., Murphy, C., Lawler, M., Fukudome, K., Smith, O., Characterization of protein C receptor expression in monocytes. *Br. J. Haematol.* 2001, 115, 408-14.

[171] Sturn, D. H., Kaneider, N. C., Feistritzer, C., Djanani, A., Fukudome, K., Wiedermann, C. J., Expression and function of the endothelial protein C receptor in human neutrophils. *Blood* 2003, 102, 1499-505.

[172] Mosnier, L. O., Griffin, J. H., Protein C anticoagulant activity in relation to anti-inflammatory and anti-apoptotic activities. *Front Biosci.* 2006, 11, 2381-99.

[173] Feistritzer, C., Mosheimer, B. A., Sturn, D. H., Riewald, M., Patsch, J. R., Wiedermann, C. J., Endothelial protein C receptor-dependent inhibition of migration of human lymphocytes by protein C involves epidermal growth factor receptor. *J. Immunol.* 2006, 176, 1019-25.

[174] Kurata, T., Hayashi, T., Yoshikawa, T., Okamoto, T., Yoshida, K., Iino, T., Uchida, A., Suzuki, K., Activated protein C stimulates osteoblast proliferation via endothelial protein C receptor. *Thromb. Res.* 2010, 125, 184-91.

[175] Nakamura, M., Gabazza, E. C., Imoto, I., Yano, Y., Taguchi, O., Horiki, N., Fukudome, K., Suzuki, K., Adachi, Y., Anti-inflammatory effect of activated protein C in gastric epithelial cells. *J. Thromb. Haemost.* 2005, 3, 2721-9.

[176] Jackson, M. T., Smith, M. M., Smith, S. M., Jackson, C. J., Xue, M., Little, C. B., Activation of cartilage matrix metalloproteinases by activated protein C. *Arthritis Rheum.* 2009, 60, 780-91.

[177] Xue, M., Campbell, D., Jackson, C. J., Protein C is an autocrine growth factor for human skin keratinocytes. *J. Biol. Chem.* 2007, 282, 13610-6.

[178] Xue, M., Smith, M. M., Little, C. B., Sambrook, P., March, L., Jackson, C. J., Activated protein C mediates a healing phenotype in cultured tenocytes. *J. Cell. Mol. Med.* 2009, 13, 749-57.

[179] Bretschneider, E., Uzonyi, B., Weber, A. A., Fischer, J. W., Pape, R., Lötzer, K., Schrör, K., Human vascular smooth muscle cells express functionally active endothelial cell protein C receptor. *Circ. Res.* 2007, 100, 255-62.

[180] Kerschen, E., Hernandez, I., Zogg, M., Jia, S., Hessner, M. J., Fernandez, J. A., Griffin, J. H., Huettner, C. S., Castellino, F. J., Weiler, H., Activated protein C targets CD8+ dendritic cells to reduce the mortality of endotoxemia in mice. *J. Clin. Invest.* 2010, 120, 3167-78.

[181] Balazs, A. B., Fabian, A. J., Esmon, C. T., Mulligan, R. C., Endothelial protein C receptor (CD201) explicitly identifies hematopoietic stem cells in murine bone marrow. *Blood* 2006, 107, 2317-21.

[182] Wang, J., Yang, L., Rezaie, A. R., Li, J., Activated protein C protects against myocardial ischemic/reperfusion injury through AMP-activated protein kinase signaling. *J. Thromb. Haemost.* 2011, 9, 1308-17.

[183] Gu, J. M., Crawley, J. T., Ferrell, G., Zhang, F., Li, W., Esmon, N. L., Esmon, C. T., Disruption of the endothelial cell protein C receptor gene

in mice causes placental thrombosis and early embryonic lethality. *J. Biol. Chem.* 2002, 277, 43335-43.

[184] Uitte de Willige, S., Van Marion, V., Rosendaal, F. R., Vos, H. L., de Visser, M. C., Bertina, R. M., Haplotypes of the EPCR gene, plasma sEPCR levels and the risk of deep venous thrombosis. *J. Thromb. Haemost.* 2004, 2, 1305-10.

[185] Simioni, P., Morboeuf, O., Tognin, G., Gavasso, S., Tormene, D., Woodhams, B., Pagnan, A., Soluble endothelial protein C receptor (sEPCR) levels and venous thromboembolism in carriers of two dysfunctional protein C variants. *Thromb. Res.* 2006, 117, 523-8.

[186] Seligsohn, U., Zivelin, A., Thrombophilia as a multigenic disorder. *Thromb. Haemost.* 1997, 78, 297-301.

[187] Zöller, B., García de Frutos, P., Hillarp, A., Dahlbäck, B., Thrombophilia as a multigenic disease. *Haematologica* 1999, 84, 59-70.

[188] Biguzzi, E., Merati, G., Liaw, P. C., Bucciarelli, P., Oganesyan, N., Qu, D., Gu, J. M., Fetiveau, R., Esmon, C. T., Mannucci, P. M., Faioni, E. M., A 23bp insertion in the endothelial protein C receptor (EPCR) gene impairs EPCR function. *Thromb. Haemost.* 2001, 86, 945-8.

[189] Biguzzi, E., Gu, J. M., Merati, G., Esmon, N. L., Esmon, C. T., Point mutations in the endothelial protein C receptor (EPCR) promoter. *Thromb. Haemost.* 2002, 87, 1085-6.

[190] Medina, P., Navarro, S., Estellés, A., España, F., Polymorphisms in the endothelial protein C receptor gene and thrombophilia. *Thromb. Haemost.* 2007, 98, 564-9.

[191] Merati, G., Biguzzi, E., Oganesyan, N., Fetiveau, R., Qu, D., Bucciarelli, P., A 23bp insertion in the endothelial protein C receptor (EPCR) gene in patients with myocardial infarction and deep vein thrombosis Supplement to the journal, *Thromb. Haemost.*, 1999 p. 507.

[192] Von Depka, M., Czwalinna, A., Eisert, R., Wermes, C., Scharrer, I., Ganser, A., Ehrenforth, S., Prevalence of a 23bp insertion in exon 3 of the endothelial cell protein C receptor gene in venous thrombophilia. *Thromb. Haemost.* 2001, 86, 1360-2.

[193] Poort, S. R., Vos, H. L., Rosendaal, F. R., Bertina, R. M., The endothelial protein C receptor (EPCR) 23 bp insert mutation and the risk of venous thrombosis. *Thromb. Haemost.* 2002, 88, 160-2.

[194] Akar, N., Gökdemir, R., Ozel, D., Akar, E., Endothelial cell protein C receptor (EPCR) gene exon III, 23 bp insertion mutation in the Turkish pediatric thrombotic patients. *Thromb. Haemost.* 2002, 88, 1068-9.

[195] Galligan, L., Livingstone, W., Mynett-Johnston, L., Smith, O. P., Prevalence of the 23bp endothelial protein C receptor (EPCR) gene insertion in the Irish population. *Thromb. Haemost.* 2002, 87, 773-4.

[196] Grossmann, R., Schwender, S., Geisen, U., Schambeck, C., Merati, G., Walter, U., CBS 844ins68, MTHFR TT677 and EPCR 4031ins23 genotypes in patients with deep-vein thrombosis. *Thromb. Res.* 2002, 107, 13-5.

[197] Franchi, F., Biguzzi, E., Cetin, I., Facchetti, F., Radaelli, T., Bozzo, M., Pardi, G., Faioni, E. M., Mutations in the thrombomodulin and endothelial protein C receptor genes in women with late fetal loss. *Br. J. Haematol.* 2001, 114, 641-6.

[198] Hermida, J., Hurtado, V., Villegas-Mendez, A., Catto, A. J., Philippou, H., Identification and characterization of a natural R96C EPCR variant. *J. Thromb. Haemost.* 2003, 1, 1850-2.

[199] Simmonds, R. E., Lane, D. A., Structural and functional implications of the intron/exon organization of the human endothelial cell protein C/ activated protein C receptor (EPCR) gene: comparison with the structure of CD1/major histocompatibility complex alpha1 and alpha2 domains. *Blood* 1999, 94, 632-41.

[200] Saposnik, B., Reny, J. L., Gaussem, P., Emmerich, J., Aiach, M., Gandrille, S., A haplotype of the EPCR gene is associated with increased plasma levels of sEPCR and is a candidate risk factor for thrombosis. *Blood* 2004, 103, 1311-8.

[201] Medina, P., Navarro, S., Estellés, A., Vayá, A., Woodhams, B., Mira, Y., Villa, P., Migaud-Fressart, M., Ferrando, F., Aznar, J., Bertina, R. M., España, F., Contribution of polymorphisms in the endothelial protein C receptor gene to soluble endothelial protein C receptor and circulating activated protein C levels, and thrombotic risk. *Thromb. Haemost.* 2004, 91, 905-11.

[202] Medina, P., Bonet, E., Navarro, S., Martos, L., Estellés, A., Ferrando, F., Vicente, V., Bertina, R. M., España, F., Effects of oral anticoagulant therapy and haplotype 1 of the endothelial protein C receptor gene on activated protein C levels. *Thromb. Haemost.* 2012, 107, 448-57.

[203] Pecheniuk, N. M., Elias, D. J., Xu, X., Griffin, J. H., Failure to validate association of gene polymorphisms in EPCR, PAR-1, FSAP and protein S Tokushima with venous thromboembolism among Californians of European ancestry. *Thromb. Haemost.* 2008, 99, 453-5.

[204] Espana, F., Zuazu, I., Vicente, V., Estellés, A., Marco, P., Aznar, J., Quantification of circulating activated protein C in human plasma by

immunoassays--enzyme levels are proportional to total protein C levels. *Thromb. Haemost.* 1996, 75, 56-61.

[205] Yamagishi, K., Cushman, M., Heckbert, S. R., Tsai, M. Y., Folsom, A. R., Lack of association of soluble endothelial protein C receptor and PROCR 6936A/G polymorphism with the risk of venous thromboembolism in a prospective study. *Br. J. Haematol.* 2009, 145, 221-6.

[206] Ireland, H., Konstantoulas, C. J., Cooper, J. A., Hawe, E., Humphries, S. E., Mather, H., Goodall, A. H., Hogwood, J., Juhan-Vague, I., Yudkin, J. S., di Minno, G., Margaglione, M., Hamsten, A., Miller, G. J., Bauer, K. A., Kim, Y. T., Stearns-Kurosawa, D. J., Kurosawa, S., EPCR Ser219 Gly: elevated sEPCR, prothrombin F1+2, risk for coronary heart disease, and increased sEPCR shedding in vitro. *Atherosclerosis* 2005, 183, 283-92.

[207] Medina, P., Navarro, S., Corral, J., Zorio, E., Roldán, V., Estellés, A., Santamaría, A., Marín, F., Rueda, J., Bertina, R. M., España, F., Groups, R. T., Endothelial protein C receptor polymorphisms and risk of myocardial infarction. *Haematologica* 2008, 93, 1358-63.

[208] Chen, X. D., Tian, L., Li, M., Jin, W., Zhang, H. K., Zheng, C. F., Relationship between endothelial cell protein C receptor gene 6936A/G polymorphisms and deep venous thrombosis. *Chin. Med. J. (Engl.)* 2011, 124, 72-5.

[209] Dennis, J., Johnson, C. Y., Adediran, A. S., de Andrade, M., Heit, J. A., Morange, P. E., Trégouët, D. A., Gagnon, F., The endothelial protein C receptor (PROCR) Ser219Gly variant and risk of common thrombotic disorders: a HuGE review and meta-analysis of evidence from observational studies. *Blood* 2012, 119, 2392-400.

[210] Qu, D., Wang, Y., Song, Y., Esmon, N. L., Esmon, C. T., The Ser219-->Gly dimorphism of the endothelial protein C receptor contributes to the higher soluble protein levels observed in individuals with the A3 haplotype. *J. Thromb. Haemost.* 2006, 4, 229-35.

[211] Saposnik, B., Lesteven, E., Lokajczyk, A., Esmon, C. T., Aiach, M., Gandrille, S., Alternative mRNA is favored by the A3 haplotype of the EPCR gene PROCR and generates a novel soluble form of EPCR in plasma. *Blood* 2008, 111, 3442-51.

[212] Ireland, H. A., Cooper, J. A., Drenos, F., Acharya, J., Mitchell, J. P., Bauer, K. A., Morrissey, J. H., Esnouf, M. P., Humphries, S. E., FVII, FVIIa, and downstream markers of extrinsic pathway activation differ by EPCR Ser219Gly variant in healthy men. *Arterioscler. Thromb. Vasc. Biol.* 2009, 29, 1968-74.

[213] Esmon, C. T., Fukudome, K., Mather, T., Bode, W., Regan, L. M., Stearns-Kurosawa, D. J., Kurosawa, S., Inflammation, sepsis, and coagulation. *Haematologica* 1999, 84, 254-9.
[214] Espana, F., Medina, P., Navarro, S., Zorio, E., Estellés, A., Aznar, J., The multifunctional protein C system. *Curr. Med. Chem. Cardiovasc. Hematol. Agents* 2005, 3, 119-31.
[215] Li, J. Y., Su, C. H., Wu, Y. J., Tien, T. Y., Hsieh, C. L., Chen, C. H., Tseng, Y. M., Shi, G. Y., Wu, H. L., Tsai, C. H., Lin, F. Y., Yeh, H. I., Therapeutic angiogenesis of human early endothelial progenitor cells is enhanced by thrombomodulin. *Arterioscler. Thromb. Vasc. Biol.* 2011, 31, 2518-25.
[216] Ikezoe, T., Yang, J., Nishioka, C., Honda, G., Furihata, M., Yokoyama, A., Thrombomodulin protects endothelial cells from a calcineurin inhibitor-induced cytotoxicity by upregulation of extracellular signal-regulated kinase/myeloid leukemia cell-1 signaling. *Arterioscler. Thromb. Vasc. Biol.* 2012, 32, 2259-70.
[217] Weiler-Guettler, H., Christie, P. D., Beeler, D. L., Healy, A. M., Hancock, W. W., Rayburn, H., Edelberg, J. M., Rosenberg, R. D., A targeted point mutation in thrombomodulin generates viable mice with a prethrombotic state. *J. Clin. Invest.* 1998, 101, 1983-91.
[218] Isermann, B., Hendrickson, S. B., Zogg, M., Wing, M., Cummiskey, M., Kisanuki, Y. Y., Yanagisawa, M., Weiler, H., Endothelium-specific loss of murine thrombomodulin disrupts the protein C anticoagulant pathway and causes juvenile-onset thrombosis. *J. Clin. Invest.* 2001, 108, 537-46.
[219] Raife, T. J., Dwyre, D. M., Stevens, J. W., Erger, R. A., Leo, L., Wilson, K. M., Fernández, J. A., Wilder, J., Kim, H. S., Griffin, J. H., Maeda, N., Lentz, S. R., Human thrombomodulin knock-in mice reveal differential effects of human thrombomodulin on thrombosis and atherosclerosis. *Arterioscler. Thromb. Vasc. Biol.* 2011, 31, 2509-17.
[220] Ishii, H., Majerus, P. W., Thrombomodulin is present in human plasma and urine. *J. Clin. Invest.* 1985, 76, 2178-81.
[221] Takano, S., Kimura, S., Ohdama, S., Aoki, N., Plasma thrombomodulin in health and diseases. *Blood* 1990, 76, 2024-9.
[222] Ohlin, A. K., Larsson, K., Hansson, M., Soluble thrombomodulin activity and soluble thrombomodulin antigen in plasma. *J. Thromb. Haemost.* 2005, 3, 976-82.
[223] Loreth, R., Seus, C., Berger, H., Albert, F., Plasma thrombomodulin concentrations in healthy persons depends on age and sex. *Supplement to the journal Ann. Hematol.*, 1997; p. 74.

[224] Amiral, J., Adam, M., Mimilla, F., Larrivaz, I., Chambrette, B., Boffa, M. C., Design and validation of a new immunoassay for soluble forms of thrombomodulin and studies on plasma. *Hybridoma* 1994, 13, 205-13.
[225] Weiler, H., Isermann, B. H., Thrombomodulin. *J. Thromb. Haemost.* 2003, 1, 1515-24.
[226] Van der Velden, P. A., Krommenhoek-Van Es, T., Allaart, C. F., Bertina, R. M., Reitsma, P. H., A frequent thrombomodulin amino acid dimorphism is not associated with thrombophilia. *Thromb. Haemost.* 1991, 65, 511-3.
[227] Ohlin, A. K., Marlar, R. A., The first mutation identified in the thrombomodulin gene in a 45-year-old man presenting with thromboembolic disease. *Blood* 1995, 85, 330-6.
[228] Medina, P., España, F., Villa, P., Vayá, A., Mira, Y., Estellés, A., Royo, M., Bertina, R., Aznar, J., The C1418T polymorphism in the thrombomodulin gene is associated with increased levels of circulating activated protein C. *Supplement to the journal Thromb. Haemost.*, 2001.
[229] Aleksic, N., Folsom, A. R., Cushman, M., Heckbert, S. R., Tsai, M. Y., Wu, K. K., Prospective study of the A455V polymorphism in the thrombomodulin gene, plasma thrombomodulin, and incidence of venous thromboembolism: the LITE Study. *J. Thromb. Haemost.* 2003, 1, 88-94.
[230] Heit, J. A., Petterson, T. M., Owen, W. G., Burke, J. P., De Andrade, M., Melton, L. J., Thrombomodulin gene polymorphisms or haplotypes as potential risk factors for venous thromboembolism: a population-based case-control study. *J. Thromb. Haemost.* 2005, 3, 710-7.
[231] Ireland, H., Kunz, G., Kyriakoulis, K., Stubbs, P. J., Lane, D. A., Thrombomodulin gene mutations associated with myocardial infarction. *Circulation* 1997, 96, 15-8.
[232] Norlund, L., Holm, J., Zöller, B., Ohlin, A. K., A common thrombomodulin amino acid dimorphism is associated with myocardial infarction. *Thromb. Haemost.* 1997, 77, 248-51.
[233] Wu, K. K., Aleksic, N., Ahn, C., Boerwinkle, E., Folsom, A. R., Juneja, H., Investigators, A. R. i. C. S. A., Thrombomodulin Ala455Val polymorphism and risk of coronary heart disease. *Circulation* 2001, 103, 1386-9.
[234] Sugiyama, S., Hirota, H., Kimura, R., Kokubo, Y., Kawasaki, T., Suehisa, E., Okayama, A., Tomoike, H., Hayashi, T., Nishigami, K., Kawase, I., Miyata, T., Haplotype of thrombomodulin gene associated

with plasma thrombomodulin level and deep vein thrombosis in the Japanese population. *Thromb. Res.* 2007, 119, 35-43.

[235] Konstantoulas, C. J., Cooper, J., Warnock, G., Miller, G. J., Humphries, S. E., Ireland, H., A combination of two common thrombomodulin gene variants (-1208-1209TTdelTT and A455V) influence risk of coronary heart disease: a prospective study in men. *Atherosclerosis* 2004, 177, 97-104.

[236] Navarro, S., Medina, P., Bonet, E., Corral, J., Martínez-Sales, V., Martos, L., Rivera, M., Roselló-Lletí, E., Alberca, I., Roldán, V., Mira, Y., Ferrando, F., Estellés, A., Vicente, V., Bertina, R. M., España, F., Association of the thrombomodulin gene c.1418C>T polymorphism with thrombomodulin levels and with venous thrombosis risk. *Arterioscler. Thromb. Vasc. Biol.* 2013, 33, 1435-40.

[237] Nakabayashi, M., Yamamoto, S., Suzuki, K., Analysis of thrombomodulin gene polymorphism in women with severe early-onset preeclampsia. *Semin. Thromb. Hemost.* 1999, 25, 473-9.

[238] Jackson, D. E., Tetaz, T. J., Salem, H. H., Mitchell, C. A., Purification and characterization of two forms of soluble thrombomodulin from human urine. *Eur. J. Biochem.* 1994, 221, 1079-87.

[239] Strandberg, K., Svensson, P. J., Ohlin, A. K., Venous thromboembolism in carriers of the Factor V Leiden mutation and in patients without known thrombophilic risk factor; prediction of recurrence and APC-PCI complex concentration and/or soluble thrombomodulin antigen and activity. *Thromb. Res.* 2007, 121, 145-51.

[240] Auro, K., Komulainen, K., Alanne, M., Silander, K., Peltonen, L., Perola, M., Salomaa, V., Thrombomodulin gene polymorphisms and haplotypes and the risk of cardiovascular events: a prospective follow-up study. *Arterioscler. Thromb. Vasc. Biol.* 2006, 26, 942-7.

[241] Van de Poel, R. H., Meijers, J. C., Rosing, J., Tans, G., Bouma, B. N., C4b-binding protein protects coagulation factor Va from inactivation by activated protein C. *Biochemistry* 2000, 39, 14543-8.

[242] Esmon, C. T., Inflammation and thrombosis. *J. Thromb. Haemost.* 2003, 1, 1343-8.

[243] Houlihan, L. M., Davies, G., Tenesa, A., Harris, S. E., Luciano, M., Gow, A. J., McGhee, K. A., Liewald, D. C., Porteous, D. J., Starr, J. M., Lowe, G. D., Visscher, P. M., Deary, I. J., Common variants of large effect in F12, KNG1, and HRG are associated with activated partial thromboplastin time. *Am. J. Hum. Genet.* 2010, 86, 626-31.

[244] Gailani, D., Renné, T., The intrinsic pathway of coagulation: a target for treating thromboembolic disease? *J. Thromb. Haemost.* 2007, 5, 1106-12.

[245] Morange, P. E., Oudot-Mellakh, T., Cohen, W., Germain, M., Saut, N., Antoni, G., Alessi, M. C., Bertrand, M., Dupuy, A. M., Letenneur, L., Lathrop, M., Lopez, L. M., Lambert, J. C., Emmerich, J., Amouyel, P., Trégouët, D. A., KNG1 Ile581Thr and susceptibility to venous thrombosis. *Blood* 2011, 117, 3692-4.

[246] Sabater-Lleal, M., Martinez-Perez, A., Buil, A., Folkersen, L., Souto, J. C., Bruzelius, M., Borrell, M., Odeberg, J., Silveira, A., Eriksson, P., Almasy, L., Hamsten, A., Soria, J. M., A genome-wide association study identifies KNG1 as a genetic determinant of plasma factor XI Level and activated partial thromboplastin time. *Arterioscler. Thromb. Vasc. Biol.* 2012, 32, 2008-16.

In: Venous Thrombosis
Editor: Caroline H. Gutmann
ISBN: 978-1-63117-293-9

Chapter 6

Genetic Risk Factors and Prevention of Venous Thromboembolism

Yu Hu and Liang Tang
Institute of Hematology, Union Hospital, Tongji Medical College,
Huazhong University of Science and Technology,
Wuhan, Hubei, China

Abstract

The annual incidence of venous thrombosis varies from 40 per 100,000 to 250 per 100,000 in different populations. Thrombosis can occur in any section of the venous system, but commonly manifests as deep vein thrombosis of the leg and pulmonary embolism. Major complications of venous thrombosis are a disabling post-thrombotic syndrome, pulmonary hypertension, and sudden death duo to a pulmonary embolism and therefore, it poses a burden on health economy. Venous thrombosis is a common clinical challenge for doctors of all disciplines, as it is a complex multicausal disease. Hereditary conditions account for ~60% of all the thrombosis incidents and a number of genetic risk factors have been identified so far. Acquired risk factors may contribute to variations within and between individuals. Diagnosis of thrombosis is not difficult with the development of imaging techniques. However, the most important steps for diagnosis are etiology analyzes and genetic tests, which are useful for assessments of duration of anticoagulant therapy and prevention for thrombosis.

1. The Pathogenesis and Risk Factors of Venous Thrombosis

Under physiological conditions, hemostasis involves the activation, adherence and aggregation of platelets and the subsequent blood coagulation that leads to the formation of fibrin clots [1]. Blood coagulation implicates a cascade activation of endogenous and exogenous coagulation factors, which results in a high local concentration of thrombins [2]. The coagulation process is regulated by multiple anticoagulation systems *in vivo*, which promptly provide feedback inhibition for unlimited coagulation amplification [3]. First, inhibitors of the tissue factor pathway may bind to the tissue factor-factor VIIa (TF-FVIIa) complex to suppress the activation of the exogenous factor X (FX); this deactivation process is elevated ten-fold by the auxiliary protein S (PS). Second, thrombin catalyzes the activation of protein C (PC), which becomes activated protein C (APC) and, in the presence of its cofactor PS, inactivates coagulation factor Va (FVa) through feedback; meanwhile, under the mutual activities of non-activated coagulation factor V (FV) and PS, APC can effectively degrade FVIIIa. Notably, thrombin itself activates PC very slowly, but the activation rate is augmented almost 1000-fold with the auxiliary effects of thrombomodulin. In addition, endothelial protein C receptors also boost the PC activation rate to a certain degree. Third, antithrombin, assisted by heparin or heparan sulfate, inhibits the activities of thrombin and coagulation factors such as FXa, FIXa and FXIa. Fourth, in the presence of cofactors of protein Z, PZ-dependent protease inhibitors can inhibit the procoagulant activity of FXa. Fifth, plasma β2-glycoprotein I directly inhibits the procoagulant activity of thrombin without affecting the anticoagulant property of thrombin-activated PC. Concurrent with the initiation of coagulation and anticoagulation systems, the fibrinolytic system in the body is also activated to generate plasmin, which clears the emerged thrombi; the plasmin level is modulated by plasminogen and its inhibitors.

In 1856, Virchow proposed three major elements of pathological thrombosis: vascular wall injury, hemodynamic changes and changes in blood components (coagulation, anticoagulation and fibrinolysis systems). Hence, any factor that affects these steps can become a risk factor for venous thrombosis. As a typical multifactorial disease, venous thrombosis is determined by multiple hereditary and acquired factors. Family-based and twin-based studies have revealed that approximately 60% of venous thromboembolism (VTE) is attributable to genetic factors [4]; these factors determine different individuals' susceptibility to VTE under the same environment or condition. Table 1 summarizes the common hereditary risk factors for venous thrombosis. Many acquired risk factors have gradually been recognized as well [22]. First, advanced age is the most common acquired risk factor for arteriovenous thrombotic diseases. Studies show that the VTE incidence in children is only 5/100,000, whereas in elderly people over 80 years old, the incidence is as high as 450 to 600/100,000; in addition, several cohort studies have indicated that individuals over 60 years old have a VTE risk significantly higher than those younger than 60 years (hazard ratio, 1.8; 95% confidence interval, 1.2-2.7).

Table 1. Common genetic risk factors for venous thrombosis

Mutations or polymorphisms	Mechanisms of venous thrombosis	Endemic population	Ref
PROC p.Arg189Trp	A missense mutation causes type II protein C (PC) deficiency and decreased PC anticoagulant activities.	Han Chinese in China	[5]
PROC p.Lys192del	A deletion mutation causes PC to lose a normal Lys residue and decreases PC anticoagulant activities.	Han Chinese in China	[6]
THBD c.–151G>T	A 5'UTR point mutation causes reduced expression of the transmembrane protein TM and a diminished rate of PC activation.	Han Chinese in China	[7]
F5 Leiden	A missense mutation of R506Q in FV causes resistance to APC inactivation.	European and American whites	[8-10]
F2 G20210A	A 3'UTR point mutation causes decreased mRNA stability and lower abundance of prothrombin.	European and American whites	[11]
PROS1 p.Lys196Glu	A missense mutation causes diminished anticoagulant activities of the PS cofactor.	Japan	[12]
Hereditary AT deficiency	Various rare mutations in *SERPINC1* decrease the expression levels or anticoagulant activity of AT.	Various populations	[13]
Hereditary PC deficiency	Various rare mutations in *PROC* decrease the expression and anticoagulant activity of PC.	Various populations	[14, 15]
Hereditary PS deficiency	Various rare mutations in *PROS1* decrease the expression level and anticoagulant activity of PS.	Various populations	[16, 17]
Hereditary TM deficiency	Various rare mutations in *THBD* decrease the expression level and anticoagulant activity of TM.	Various populations [d]	[18, 19]
rs8176719 polymorphism	Determines whether plasma FVIII and vWF levels are significantly elevated in O type or non-O type blood (using the ABO system).	Various populations	[20, 21]

The venous thrombotic state in individuals of advanced age is mainly associated with reduced vascular endothelial functions. Second, complex trauma and surgery (especially neurosurgery and orthopedic surgery) are both high-risk factors for VTE (odds ratio, OR: ~10); patients have a VTE incidence greater than 50% if anticoagulant prophylaxis is not provided. The thrombotic risk of surgery and trauma is mainly related to the release of tissue factors, the increased abundance of acute phase proteins (e.g., FVIII and fibrinogen) and limb immobilization. Third, malignancy is an independent risk factor for VTE. MEGA studies revealed that cancer increased the VTE risk by nearly a factor of seven. Among various malignancies, hematological cancers have the highest thrombotic risk (OR: ~28.0), followed by lung cancer and gastrointestinal cancer. The underlying mechanisms whereby malignancies lead to venous thrombosis primarily include the release of procoagulant substances and tissue factors, diminished AT levels, the mechanical pressure and blood pressure blockage from tumors, reduced activity, chemotherapy and radiotherapy and central venous catheterization. Fourth, patients with VTE history have a five-fold increase in thrombotic risk and a three-year recurrence rate of 15 to 25%.

In addition, individuals with a thrombotic family history have variously elevated VTE risks. Fifth, pregnancy puerperium, oral contraceptives and estrogen replacement therapy increases levels of procoagulant factors, including FVII, FVIII, FX, fibrinogen and von Willebrand factor (vWF) and decreases the level of free PS, which also leads to acquired venous thrombosis. Sixth, a sustained presence of antiphospholipid antibodies in the body is also an arteriovenous thrombotic risk factor frequently found in certain populations. Common antiphospholipid antibodies mainly comprise anti-cardiolipin antibodies, lupus anticoagulant (LA) and anti-β2GPI antibodies. Anti-cardiolipin antibodies are merely a weak VTE risk factor (OR: ~1.1); LA and anti-β2GPI antibodies are the main antibodies causing hypercoagulation (OR: 6~11), as relevant studies have revealed. Noticeably, the specific structure and constituents of LA are currently unclear, and the existence of LA is only inferred from the laboratory examination of anticoagulant compounds in blood samples.

Using a statistical case-control study model, it has been revealed that after correcting the variable of anti-β2GPI antibodies, the LA-dependent VTE risk disappeared. This finding suggests that further investigation is needed to explore whether anti-β2GPI antibodies are a major type of LA. Seventh, elements causing long-term limb immobilization directly influence hemodynamics and cause hypercoagulation; therefore, they are recognized as

VTE risk factors. For example, it has been reported that long-distance flights are correlated with a two- to four-fold increase in the occurrence of VTE. Nevertheless, the definition of "long-term immobilization" is not currently standardized and can range from four hours to three days. Eighth, excessive obesity (BMI>30 kg/m^2) increases the risk of developing VTE by approximately a factor of two, which may be explained by markedly elevated levels of FVIII and FIX in obese individuals. Ninth, patients with chronic renal insufficiency and nephrotic syndrome have a significantly increased concentration of multiple coagulation factors in the blood and a relative deficiency of low-molecular anticoagulant proteins, such as AT, and therefore have hypercoagulation. In addition, long-term administration of glucocorticoids and central venous catheterization can further augment the thrombotic risk. Tenth, some acute diseases, such as acute myocardial infarction, acute heart failure (NYHA Class III or IV), acute infectious diseases (lower extremity cellulitis), acute respiratory diseases (respiratory failure), acute rheumatic diseases, acute stroke and autoimmune diseases are also acquired VTE risk factors and may be associated with the release of inflammatory cytokines and procoagulant molecules.

2. Clinical Manifestations, Diagnosis and Etiology Screening of Venous Thrombosis and Questions for Consideration

2.1. Clinical Manifestations and Diagnosis of Venous Thrombosis

Venous thrombosis is characterized by the formation of thrombotic structures and the development of thromboembolic diseases; most cases are venous thromboembolism (VTE), which includes deep-vein thrombosis (DVT) and pulmonary thromboembolism (PTE). For hemodynamic reasons, DVT often occurs in the lower extremities; its main clinical manifestations are pain in the affected limbs, swelling and varicose veins. Rapidly developing and extensively distributed DVT in the lower limbs may be accompanied by periphlebitis and oppression lesions in the pelvic veins and the lymphatic system, which give rise to phlegmasia alba dolens, or "white leg"; the disease may further progress to impact the arterial blood supply system and cause gangrene, thereby leading to phlegmasia cerulea dolens, or "blue leg". Moreover, recurrent DVT tends to post-thrombosis syndrome (PTS), in which the affected limbs display various levels of swelling and varicose veins, persistent skin ulcers and even dysfunction. PTE may occur after lower extremity DVT or independently and can have a mortality rate of 33% if timely diagnosis and intervention are not provided. Most PTE patients do not display the typical triad of "chest pain, hemoptysis and dyspnea". Hence, the key to improving diagnosis is to better understand the disease; whenever a patient shows chest tightness, shortness of breath, fainting and symptoms of coronary heart disease, the possibility of PTE should be considered.

For patients with hereditary venous thrombosis (e.g., PC deficiency, PS deficiency and AT deficiency), a thrombus can also implicate some rare sites, such as thrombosis in the cerebral venous sinus, the mesenteric vein, the upper limb (axillary vein), the renal vein and the portal vein.

Homozygous hereditary venous thrombosis (e.g., homozygous PC deficiency) may cause extensive and very large thrombosis and purpura fulminans in newborn babies. In addition, venous thrombosis can also result in arterial thrombotic diseases, including ischemic stroke, acute myocardial infarction and extremity artery thrombosis. Some types of venous thrombosis (PC deficiency, PS deficiency, *F5* Leiden, TM deficiency, antiphospholipid syndrome) can also cause habitual abortion, fetal growth retardation and stillbirth.

For patients with a putative VTE diagnosis, a convincing conclusion can be obtained by integrating the thrombotic clinical manifestations combined with plasma D-dimer levels and objective laboratory examinations. The D-dimer level is often detected using enzyme-linked immunosorbent assay (ELISA) because acute VTE patients have a plasma D-dimer level of 0.5 mg/L above the normal upper threshold value. This method has a low specificity because advanced ages (>80 years), infections, tumors and tissue necrosis can all cause an increased D-dimer level; on the other hand, this assay is very sensitive (>99%), and acute VTE always results in D-dimer elevation. Therefore, aberrant examination results do not necessarily indicate VTE, whereas normal results can exclude VTE. To diagnose DVT, color Doppler ultrasonography has a high sensitivity and specificity (~95%) and is therefore a common auxiliary test. Although venography is a gold standard, it is invasive and is therefore only used in highly suspected cases in which ultrasonography does not reveal any thrombotic sign. As for PTE, spiral CT pulmonary angiography has gradually become a top diagnostic method; as an auxiliary approach, it yields a sensitivity of 82 to 99% and a specificity of 92 to 96% for central PTE.

2.2. Etiology Screening of Venous Thrombosis and Questions for Consideration

It is not difficult to diagnose thrombosis using currently available auxiliary methods. A more important diagnostic purpose for venous thrombosis is to identify the etiology and contributing factors. Etiology screening for venous thrombosis has a pivotal clinical significance [23-25].

The first question to ask is which patients need further screening? Given the multitude of thrombotic risk factors, there are numerous laboratory tests; a comprehensive screening will aggravate patients' economic burden, and abnormal results will intensify the patient's mental stress. Therefore, the decision about which patients need venous thrombotic screening remains controversial, and elaborate consideration is needed. In general, if one of the following signs is identified, the patient should receive further risk factor screening for venous thrombosis: 1) ischemic stroke, acute myocardial infarction or VTE onset age <45 years; 2) recurrent arteriovenous thrombosis without apparent cause; 3) unusual sites of venous thrombosis (e.g., thrombosis in the axillary vein or mesenteric vein); 4) family history of VTE; 5) occurrence of VTE with no apparent causes or with only weak acquired factors (pregnancy, puerperium, oral administration of contraceptives, estrogen replacement therapy, prolonged immobility); 6) visceral vein thrombosis or purpura fulminans in newborn babies; 7) recurrent miscarriage or stillbirth; 8) skin necrosis after oral administration of warfarin.

The next question is which risk factors for venous thrombosis should be screened. There are differences in genetic background among races or ethnic groups, and common venous thrombotic causes often differ among countries and regions. In this regard, it is necessary to first determine the common venous thrombotic risk factors in a particular population. Correspondingly, screening can be performed in the order of likeliness for the factors that may contribute to the disease. For example, the polymorphism of *F5* Leiden and *F2* G20210A are common in white populations, but are extremely rare in Asia; thus, the examination is not needed in Asian countries. A relevant point to consider is whether the remaining tests in a screening battery should be completed once an abnormality has been identified in a screening. It has been increasingly supported that screening for venous thrombosis ought to be as complete as possible, especially for patients without apparent etiology or with recurrent VTE. If initial findings are insufficient to explain recurrent thrombotic manifestations, the possibility of multiple contributing factors should be considered and tested. Actually, many clinically identified recurrent VTE patients have joint defects (e.g., joint hereditary PC-AT deficiency) [26]. Another reason to comprehensively screen for venous thrombosis is that different tests exhibit varied sensitivity to certain genetic deficiencies. For example, the gene polymorphism *PROC* p.Lys192del is a common mutation in venous thrombosis in Chinese population. When heterozygous individuals are examined for plasma PC activity, the chromogenic substrate method generates perfectly normal results, whereas the coagulation test, which is almost obsolete, is able to reveal the reduced anticoagulant activity of PC [27]. In addition, if no aberrant result is identified in routine screening tests [28-31], rare etiologies of venous thrombosis may be investigated, including hereditary dysfibrinogenemia, abnormal plasminogen and elevated levels of FIX or FXI.

3. Treatment and Prevention of Venous Thrombosis

3.1. Treatment of Venous Thrombosis

3.1.1. Thrombolytic Treatment

Approximately 5% of PTE patients display signs of unstable hemodynamics, manifesting a heart rate greater than 100 beats/min and a systolic blood pressure below 90 mmHg. These patients need immediate thrombolytic treatment. Moreover, if patients do not show improvement in PTE after aggressive anticoagulation, thrombolysis also needs to be considered.

With the exception of these conditions, thrombolysis is not recommended for the majority of PTE patients because under the conditions of venous thrombosis, thrombolysis is not more effective than anticoagulation but carries a significantly increased bleeding risk. Furthermore, extensive and critical acute iliac vein thrombosis with a complete occlusion may also be considered for thrombolysis assisted by appropriate anticoagulation.

One common thrombolytic drug is tissue-type plasminogen activator (t-PA) alteplase; 100 mg of the drug is intravenously administered within 2 hours, and the emergency protocol is to inject 0.6 mg/kg within 15 minutes.

After the completion of a thrombolytic treatment, activated partial thromboplastin time (APTT) should be monitored; when APTT drops to twice the normal upper threshold, heparin anticoagulation is started. A main side effect of the drug is bleeding; therefore, the contraindications for thrombolytic treatment mostly comprise a history of hemorrhagic stroke, ischemic stroke within six months, intracranial space-occupying lesion surgery or severe trauma within two weeks.

3.1.2. Surgical Treatment

If a patient requires emergency thrombolysis but has contraindications or experiences failed thrombolytic treatment, surgical thrombectomy is needed. However, the few available clinical reports are insufficient to determine whether the surgical approach has a better efficacy or a lower post-treatment PTS occurrence rate than anticoagulation does. Moreover, acute limb ischemia caused by arterial thrombosis also requires surgical thrombectomy, which yields a better outcome than peripheral arterial thrombolysis does.

3.1.3. Anticoagulant Treatment

Heparin is an initial anticoagulant drug for acute VTE. Its main anticoagulant mechanism is to assist antithrombin in suppressing the activities of FXa and thrombin, although heparin itself has no enzymatic activity. Because anticoagulation can be quickly and completely neutralized by protamine sulfate, the compound is predominantly used in patients with hemorrhagic risk (e.g., those who have experienced massive hemorrhage or undergone surgery), unstable hemodynamics resulting from PTE or extensive DVT or those are being considered for thrombolysis or surgical thrombectomy.

Because severe patients have reduced subcutaneous blood perfusion, intravenous injection of unfractionated heparin (UFH) has a better efficacy than the subcutaneous administration of low molecular-weight heparin [32]. Low molecular-weight heparin, fondaparinux sodium and new oral anticoagulants may accumulate in the bodies of renal failure patients (creatinine clearance rate <20 ml/min); therefore, unfractionated heparin is also recommended. Table 2 summarizes the basic applications of heparin and other anticoagulants. It should be noted that there are currently two regimens: one is to use a loading dose of 5000 U followed by 1000 U/h; the other is to use an 80-U/Kg intravenous injection followed by a maintenance dose of 18 U/kg/h. Although clinical trials have revealed that the latter yielded a lower VTE recurrence rate and lower hemorrhagic risk, the results were not statistically significant and could not lead to the conclusion that the latter was superior. Consequently, both regimens are appropriate. Heparin anticoagulation requires monitoring APTT to ensure that the plasma anti-FXa level reaches 0.3-0.7 U/mL.

Table 2. Common anticoagulant drugs for treating VTE

Anticoagulation drugs	Recommended usage	Monitoring of coagulant activity
Heparin	Loading dose at 80 U/kg, maintenance dose at 18 U/kg/h and continuous intravenous infusion, or 17,500 U subcutaneous injection, twice every day	APTT extended by one-and-a-half to two-fold Plasma anti-FXa levels reached 0.3-0.7 U/ml
Low MW heparin		
Dalteparin	200 U/kg subcutaneous injection, once every day	No monitoring
Enoxaparin	1.5 mg/kg subcutaneous injection, once every day	No monitoring
Argatroban	Continuous intravenous infusion at 2 μg/kg/min	APTT extended one-and-a-half to three-fold
Fondaparinux sodium	Body weight <50 kg, 5 mg subcutaneous injection once daily Body weight 50-100 kg, 7.5 mg subcutaneous injection once daily Body weight >100 kg, 10 mg subcutaneous injection once daily	No monitoring
Rivaroxaban	15 mg oral administration twice daily	No monitoring
Warfarin	3-4.5 mg/d oral administration, and 2-8 mg/d oral maintenance administration for 3-6 months	PT, INR[a] 2-3

a: INR, international normalized ratio.

Low molecular-weight heparin (LMWH) has the advantages of low hemorrhagic risk, no need for coagulation testing and low occurrence of heparin-induced thrombocytopenic purpura; consequently, it is more widely used than regular, unfractionated heparin. It also has an anticoagulation mechanism that assists antithrombin to suppress the activities of coagulation factors, and it has a stronger inhibitory effect on FXa than on thrombin. Noticeably, treatment in the past required LMWH to be administered once every 12 hours; however, clinical trials have demonstrated that subcutaneous injection once daily has equivalent VTE-preventative effects and safety parameters (e.g., in terms of hemorrhage and mortality) as administration twice daily. Therefore, the regimen of once per day has been recommended because of its convenience. Furthermore, once LMWH treatment yields stable conditions, no surveillance of coagulation is needed; thus, it is suitable for VTE outpatients. Studies have revealed that LMWH yielded a six-month recurrence rate (OR: 0.68; 95% CI: 0.48-0.97) and hemorrhagic risk (OR: 0.57; 95% CI: 0.39-0.83) that were both significantly lower than those of unfractionated heparin.

Fondaparinux sodium is a synthetized specific FXa inhibitor. Its coagulation-counteracting effect is also dependent on the physiological anticoagulant AT [33]. Although no relevant large-scale, random, controlled trial has been officially published, the drug has been proposed as a top anticoagulation choice for patients with a history of heparin-induced thrombocytopenia (HIT). In addition, two large-scale clinical trials revealed that fondaparinux sodium showed efficacy and safety comparable to those of LMWH and unfractionated heparin for DVT and PTE treatment.

Rivaroxaban is a novel oral FXa inhibitor. Clinical trials indicated that for the treatment of VTE, oral administration of the drug in conjunction with vitamin K antagonists showed efficacy (recurrence rate) and hemorrhagic risk equivalent to that of LMWH administration in conjunction with vitamin K antagonists. The drug reaches its peak plasma concentration 2.5 to 4 hours after administration and has a half-life of 6 to 9 hours.

3.1.4. Vitamin K Antagonists

Warfarin is a common oral anticoagulant; its mechanism is to suppress the activity of vitamin K epoxide reductase in liver mitochondria, whereby the activities of various vitamin K-dependent coagulation factors (FII, FVII, FIX and FX) are inhibited. Because the main anticoagulant proteins PC, PS and PZ in plasma also depend on vitamin K to function normally, the clinical treatment of VTE requires initial heparinization to fully restrain the activities of coagulation factors before overlapping or single oral administration of warfarin is provided. Otherwise, venous thrombosis patients with PS or PC deficiency may experience aggravated thrombotic symptoms or even warfarin-induced skin necrosis [34]. The anticoagulant effects of warfarin are influenced by genetic factors, age, race, diet and concurrent drug use; thus, the therapeutic anticoagulation plan should be determined individually. The treatment intensity ought to be monitored to keep INR at 2 to 3 because higher INR values resulting from more intense anticoagulation do not improve outcomes but do increase hemorrhagic risk. When a patient has achieved INR stability, anticoagulation is continued to keep the INR value between 0.1 and 0.5. This treatment dose is maintained for two weeks before the coagulation is rechecked.

3.1.5. Inferior Vena Cava Filter

The goal of filter placement is to prevent pulmonary embolisms caused by DVT thrombi that are shed from the lower extremities [35]. A large clinical trial examining patients with DVTs in the proximal lower extremities compared individuals who received the filter with their counterparts without the filter. The results showed that the former group had significantly lower PTE occurrence 12 days after the initial VTE events compared with the non-filtered subjects (OR: 0.22; 95% CI: 0.05-0.90). However, the filter-treated individuals had a significantly higher VTE recurrence rate (OR: 1.87; 95% CI: 1.10-3.20) two years later; the two groups exhibited overall monitoring parameters that were statistically indistinguishable at the end of the eight-year follow-up. Hence, an inferior vena cava filter is only recommended for individuals who meet the following clinical criteria: 1) patients with proximal DVT or PTE; 2) after aggressive anticoagulation treatment, patients show no improvement in VTE or even show disease progression, or have a contraindication that causes severe hemorrhage.

3.1.6. Compression Stockings

All patients with lower extremity DVT may start wearing compression stockings two weeks after the onset of the disease and may continue to do so for at least two years to prevent PTS.

3.2. Prevention of Venous Thrombosis and Questions to be Addressed

Patients with venous thrombosis have a tendency to form thrombi. When they start treatment after the occurrence of thrombotic diseases, the implicated vessels and organs have already been damaged at various levels. Hence, the emphasis of venous thrombosis management should be early diagnosis and prevention. The prevention of venous thrombosis has two aspects: to avoid recurrence in VTE patients and to prevent VTE occurrence in asymptomatic population.

3.2.1. Prevention of VTE Recurrence

Key questions to be addressed are which patients require prevention after onset of VTE, with what measures and for how long. Typically, when patients receive the standard anticoagulation, they have already taken oral warfarin to prevent VTE recurrence. Nevertheless, for patients with venous thrombotic risk factors that are long-term (e.g., malignancies) or perpetual (genetic lesions), regular treatment for three to six months is not adequate to effectively prevent VTE recurrence, and an extension of anticoagulation is needed. Alternatively, for patients who developed the disease as a result of casual acquired factors (e.g., orthopedic surgery), inappropriate treatment extension is not only meaningless from a preventative standpoint but also increases the hemorrhagic risk. Therefore, it is necessary to identify high-risk, recurrent individuals based on venous thrombotic risk factors and to establish the anticoagulation treatment time. The available literature recommends that patients with the following conditions should extend their anticoagulation treatment by six to 18 months: 1) malignancies; 2) plasma D-dimer level greater than twice the normal upper limit one month after treatment termination; and 3) temporally unavoidable risk factors, such as hormone therapy. In addition, the following factors are indicators for long-term, sustained treatment: 1) VTE in rare locations; 2) more than two VTE recurrences; 3) the persistent existence of antiphospholipid antibodies; and 4) homozygous genetic defects (e.g., homozygous *PROS1* mutation) or joint defects (e.g., AT-PC defect). To prevent recurrence, in addition to a medication-based approach, public health education is also needed to warn people to avoid acquired risk factors (e.g., smoking, obesity and a sedentary lifestyle). Notably, it is currently recommended that patients with malignancies continue full-dose LMWH anticoagulation for one month, followed by 75%-dose LMWH anticoagulation for five months after the initial heparin treatment, instead of switching to oral warfarin because switching to warfarin carries significantly higher recurrence rate and hemorrhagic risk. Another scenario to avoid when using warfarin for treatment and prevention is pregnancy because the drug may cause fetal defects. Therefore, LMWH anticoagulation cannot be terminated until the end of puerperium with a duration of no less than six months. Furthermore, clinical trials have shown that new types of oral anticoagulants (e.g., rivaroxaban) generate efficacy and safety results that are superior to or are not inferior to those of warfarin for preventing VTE and the recurrence of ischemia stroke, with the advantage of not requiring coagulation monitoring. The new oral anticoagulants are more convenient for preventing venous thrombosis, but they are also more expensive than older treatments.

3.2.2. Preventing VTE in the Asymptomatic Population

Another question to consider is whether individuals with venous thrombotic risks but no formed thrombus need preventative anticoagulation medication. For surgical and orthopedic patients, the answer is definitely "yes"; without anticoagulant prevention, these patients have a VTE occurrence rate of 50% or greater. A previous study reported that 42% of the hospitalized patients in a department of internal medicine were on the brink of VTE occurrence. Unfortunately, little attention has been paid to VTE prevention in these patients, and whether they need anticoagulation also remains unsettled. Studies have revealed that the population with heterozygous *F5* Leiden have an annual VTE occurrence rate below 1%, whereas warfarin prevention yields an annual massive hemorrhage rate of 1 to 2%. Hence, thorough consideration is needed to address the questions of whether hospitalized individuals with venous thrombotic risk but no VTE symptoms need preventative treatment, and if so, with what measures.

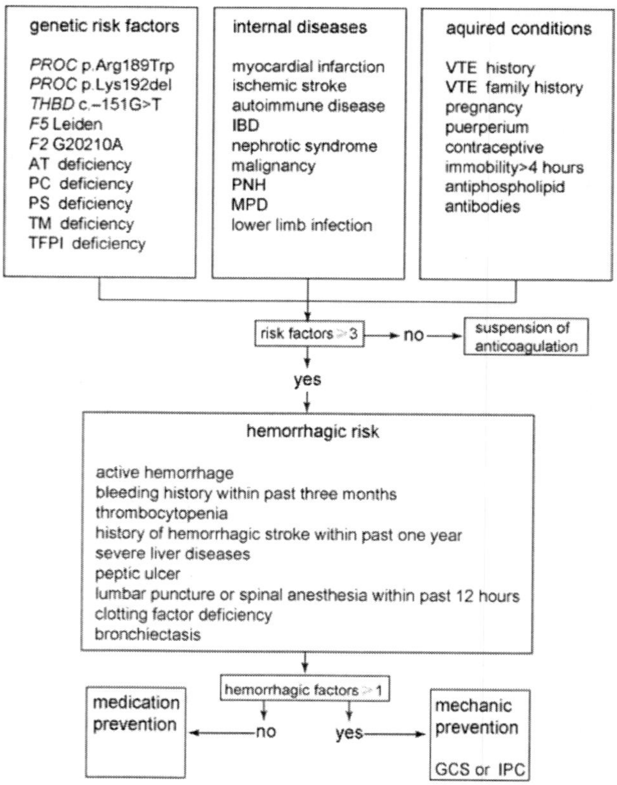

Figure 1. The VTE prevention and evaluation process for hospitalized patients in the Department of Internal Medicine. IBD: inflammatory bowel disease; MPD: myeloproliferative disorders; GCS: Graded compression stockings; IPC: Intermittent pneumatic compression devices.

Although a common solution has not yet been obtained, a preventative plan can be made based on the common hereditary, acquired risk factors for venous thrombosis, the possibility of hypercoagulation and the hemorrhagic risk in hospitalized individuals. Figure 1 gives a simple illustration of the evaluation process, which needs further improvement.

This evaluation flowchart analyzes common VTE factors and hemorrhagic risk factors, has sufficient generality and can easily be clinically implemented. Its drawback is that it discriminates among various venous thrombotic risk factors without taking the relative risk level of individual factors into account. A better evaluation method is to score all factors and weight their VTE risks. Clearly, more clinical studies are needed to facilitate a more reliable evaluation method.

References

[1] Flinterman LE, van Hylckama Vlieg A, Cannegieter SC, Rosendaal FR. Long-term survival in a large cohort of patients with venous thrombosis: incidence and predictors. *PLoS Med.* 2012;9(1):e1001155.

[2] Dahlback B. Advances in understanding pathogenic mechanisms of thrombophilic disorders. *Blood.* 2008;112(1):19-27.

[3] Reitsma PH, Versteeg HH, Middeldorp S. Mechanistic view of risk factors for venous thromboembolism. *Arterioscler. Thromb. Vasc. Biol.* 2012; 32(3):563-568.

[4] Souto JC, Almasy L, Borrell M, et al. Genetic susceptibility to thrombosis and its relationship to physiological risk factors: the GAIT study. Genetic Analysis of Idiopathic Thrombophilia. *Am. J. Hum. Genet.* 2000; 67(6):1452-1459.

[5] Tang L, Guo T, Yang R, et al. Genetic background analysis of protein C deficiency demonstrates a recurrent mutation associated with venous thrombosis in Chinese population. *PLoS One.* 2012;7(4):e35773.

[6] Tang L, Lu X, Yu JM, et al. PROC c.574_576del polymorphism: a common genetic risk factor for venous thrombosis in the Chinese population. *J. Thromb. Haemost.* 2012;10(10):2019-2026.

[7] Tang L, Wang HF, Lu X, et al. Common genetic risk factors for venous thrombosis in the Chinese population. *Am. J. Hum. Genet.* 2013; 92(2): 177-187.

[8] Dahlback B, Carlsson M, Svensson PJ. Familial thrombophilia due to a previously unrecognized mechanism characterized by poor anticoagulant

response to activated protein C: prediction of a cofactor to activated protein C. *Proc. Natl. Acad. Sci. U S A.* 1993; 90(3):1004-1008.
[9] Bertina RM, Koeleman BP, Koster T, et al. Mutation in blood coagulation factor V associated with resistance to activated protein C. *Nature.* 1994; 369(6475):64-67.
[10] Shen MC, Lin JS, Tsay W. High prevalence of antithrombin III, protein C and protein S deficiency, but no factor V Leiden mutation in venous thrombophilic Chinese patients in Taiwan. *Thromb. Res.* 1997; 87(4): 377-385.
[11] Poort SR, Rosendaal FR, Reitsma PH, Bertina RM. A common genetic variation in the 3'-untranslated region of the prothrombin gene is associated with elevated plasma prothrombin levels and an increase in venous thrombosis. *Blood.* 1996; 88(10): 3698-3703.
[12] Kimura R, Honda S, Kawasaki T, et al. Protein S-K196E mutation as a genetic risk factor for deep vein thrombosis in Japanese patients. *Blood.* 2006; 107(4):1737-1738.
[13] Luxembourg B, Delev D, Geisen C, et al. Molecular basis of antithrombin deficiency. *Thromb. Haemost.* 2011; 105(4):635-646.
[14] Gandrille S, Aiach M. Identification of mutations in 90 of 121 consecutive symptomatic French patients with a type I protein C deficiency. The French INSERM Network on Molecular Abnormalities Responsible for Protein C and Protein S deficiencies. *Blood.* 1995; 86(7):2598-2605.
[15] Mahmoodi BK, Brouwer JL, Ten Kate MK, et al. A prospective cohort study on the absolute risks of venous thromboembolism and predictive value of screening asymptomatic relatives of patients with hereditary deficiencies of protein S, protein C or antithrombin. *J. Thromb. Haemost.* 2010; 8(6):1193-1200.
[16] Zhu T, Ding Q, Bai X, et al. Normal ranges and genetic variants of antithrombin, protein C and protein S in the general Chinese population. Results of the Chinese Hemostasis Investigation on Natural Anticoagulants Study I Group. *Haematologica.* 2011; 96(7):1033-1040.
[17] Caspers M, Pavlova A, Driesen J, et al. Deficiencies of antithrombin, protein C and protein S - practical experience in genetic analysis of a large patient cohort. *Thromb. Haemost.* 2012; 108(2):247-257.
[18] Kunz G, Ireland HA, Stubbs PJ, Kahan M, Coulton GC, Lane DA. Identification and characterization of a thrombomodulin gene mutation coding for an elongated protein with reduced expression in a kindred with myocardial infarction. *Blood.* 2000;95(2):569-576.

[19] Lobato RL, White WD, Mathew JP, et al. Thrombomodulin gene variants are associated with increased mortality after coronary artery bypass surgery in replicated analyses. *Circulation.* 2011; 124(11 Suppl): S143-148.

[20] Morelli VM, De Visser MC, Vos HL, Bertina RM, Rosendaal FR. ABO blood group genotypes and the risk of venous thrombosis: effect of factor V Leiden. *J. Thromb. Haemost.* 2005; 3(1):183-185.

[21] Reilly MP, Li M, He J, et al. Identification of ADAMTS7 as a novel locus for coronary atherosclerosis and association of ABO with myocardial infarction in the presence of coronary atherosclerosis: two genome-wide association studies. *Lancet.* 2011; 377(9763):383-392.

[22] Anderson FA, Jr., Spencer FA. Risk factors for venous thromboembolism. *Circulation.* 2003;107(23 Suppl 1): I9-16.

[23] Baglin T, Gray E, Greaves M, et al. Clinical guidelines for testing for heritable thrombophilia. *Br. J. Haematol.* 2010; 149(2):209-220.

[24] Bates SM, Greer IA, Middeldorp S, Veenstra DL, Prabulos AM, Vandvik PO. VTE, thrombophilia, antithrombotic therapy, and pregnancy: Antithrombotic Therapy and Prevention of Thrombosis, 9th ed: American College of Chest Physicians Evidence-Based Clinical Practice Guidelines. *Chest.* 2012;141(2 Suppl):e691S-736S.

[25] Kyrle PA, Eichinger S. Deep vein thrombosis. *Lancet.* 2005; 365(9465): 1163-1174.

[26] Mahasandana C, Suvatte V, Marlar RA, Manco-Johnson MJ, Jacobson LJ, Hathaway WE. Neonatal purpura fulminans associated with homozygous protein S deficiency. *Lancet.* 1990; 335(8680):61-62.

[27] Bounameaux H, Rosendaal FR. Venous thromboembolism: why does ethnicity matter? *Circulation.* 2011; 123(20):2189-2191.

[28] Faioni EM, Hermida J, Rovida E, et al. Type II protein C deficiency: identification and molecular modelling of two natural mutants with low anticoagulant and normal amidolytic activity. *Br. J. Haematol.* 2000; 108(2): 265-271.

[29] Ballard RB, Marques MB. Pathology consultation on the laboratory evaluation of thrombophilia: when, how, and why. *Am. J. Clin. Pathol.* 2012; 137(4):553-560.

[30] Liberti G, Bertina RM, Rosendaal FR. Hormonal state rather than age influences cut-off values of protein S: reevaluation of the thrombotic risk associated with protein S deficiency. *Thromb. Haemost.* 1999; 82(3): 1093-1096.

[31] Baglin T, Gray E, Greaves M, et al. Clinical guidelines for testing for heritable thrombophilia. *Br. J. Haematol.* 2010; 149(2):209-220.
[32] Raschke RA, Reilly BM, Guidry JR, Fontana JR, Srinivas S. The weight-based heparin dosing nomogram compared with a "standard care" nomogram. A randomized controlled trial. *Ann. Intern. Med.* 1993; 119(9):874-881.
[33] Warkentin TE, Pai M, Sheppard JI, Schulman S, Spyropoulos AC, Eikelboom JW. Fondaparinux treatment of acute heparin-induced thrombocytopenia confirmed by the serotonin-release assay: a 30-month, 16-patient case series. *J. Thromb. Haemost.* 2011; 9(12):2389-2396.
[34] Schulman S, Melinyshyn A, Ennis D, Rudd-Scott L. Single-dose adjustment versus no adjustment of warfarin in stably anticoagulated patients with an occasional international normalized ratio (INR) out of range. *Thromb. Res.* 2010;125(5):393-397.
[35] Eight-year follow-up of patients with permanent vena cava filters in the prevention of pulmonary embolism: the PREPIC (Prevention du Risque d'Embolie Pulmonaire par Interruption Cave) randomized study. *Circulation.* 2005; 112(3):416-422.

In: Venous Thrombosis
Editor: Caroline H. Gutmann
ISBN: 978-1-63117-293-9

Chapter 7

The Prevalence of the C677T Polymorphism of the Methylenetetrahydrofolate Reductase (rs 1801133) and Classic Risk Factors in Costa Rican Women with Thrombotic Events

Lizbeth Salazar-Sánchez[1,*], Daniel Murillo[1,2,†], Juan Porras[1,3,‡], Esteban Arrieta[1,§], Mayra Cartin[1,±] and Alexander Parajeles[1,4,€]

[1]Research Centre in Hematology and Related Diseases (CIHATA)
Universidad de Costa Rica, San Juan de Dios Hospital,
San José, Costa Rica

* Research Centre in Hematology and Related Diseases CIHATA-Universidad de Costa Rica, San Juan de Dios Hospital, P.O. Box 10634-1000, San José, Costa Rica; Tel: (506) 8381-7500, Fax: (506) 2222-1385; E-mail: lizbeth.salazar@gmail.com

† Tel (506) 2222-1385; E-mail: dmurillo@medicos.cr

‡ Tel (506) 2222-1385; E-mail: jporrasp@gmail.com

§ Tel. (506) 2222-1385

± E-mail: mayra.cartin@ucr.ac.cr.

€ Tel. (506) 2222-1385; E-mail: aparajeles@yahoo.com.

[2]Internal Medicine Department, San Juan de Dios Hospital,
San José, Costa Rica
[3]Pathology Department, San Juan de Dios Hospital,
San José, Costa Rica
[4]Neurology Department, San Juan de Dios Hospital,
San José, Costa Rica

Abstract

Thrombotic diseases develop as the result of multiple interactions between non-genetic and genetic risk factors. The known atherogenic risk factors played an important role as predictors in the development of the thrombotic diseases in the present female case-control study. The most important non-genetic risk factors found among the female patients are: age, hypercholesterolemia, DM, use of oral contraception, obesity, and fibrinogen levels. Moreover, the stratified effect of some of these factors according to the age of the patients is relevant for clinical risk assessment. Associations between the risk of venous thrombosis (VT) and genetic polymorphisms have been established. Some of these polymorphisms are highly prevalent in Caucasians, but there is a significant geographic variation in their prevalence among different populations. The MTHFR C677T (rs1801133), are analyses in females with stroke, venous thrombosis and myocardial infarction in a case-control study. The C677TMTHFR mutation were detected in 149 patients and 113 controls (P=0,001). In the present study, the results showed that hypercholesterolemia, diabetes mellitus, and elevated levels of fibrinogen were present in the younger group as risks factors. Family history of thrombotic event (TE) was statistically significantly associated among the older female group. Median values of total fibrinogen were significantly higher in the cases compared with the control group. The small numbers of carriers of these risk factors require a note of caution on any conclusion. The present data suggest that MTHFR C677T genotype may be an important factor in the life of female patients at risk of developing TE or cardiovascular disease, p=0,001 between cases and controls groups. Folic acid supplementation of foods is necessary (and mandatory in Costa Rica) before and during women's reproductive phase. However, our data presented suggest that a case for efforts to ensure a good intake of this vitamin in the postmenopausal phase. Especially if the high prevalence of the MTHFR 677T homozygosity and of classic risk factors in the Costa Rican population are taken into account. Further studies with more patients are necessary for final conclusions for these interactions to be drawn.

Introduction

The general definition of thrombotic event (TE) refers to a clot large enough to cause occlusion of flow through a blood vessel, either arterial or venous. The clinical manifestations of this event depend on the site of occlusion. Several pathophysiologic mechanisms have been described for this condition, such as intrinsic blood vessel involvement (most frequent), later participation of the humoral components of the primary coagulation pathways, and less frequent involvement of platelet activation.

The most common type of TE is acute coronary syndrome a component of coronary atherosclerotic disease causing ischemic heart disease, which is the leading cause of death in Costa Rica (Araya & Guzman, 2004) and, consequently, a significant proportion of the TE diagnoses in hospitals. Therefore, any effort to elucidate and identify factors that may intervene in primary and secondary prevention of this condition is clearly justified.

Thrombophilia is a disorder hemostasis where a tendency for the thrombosis in veins or arteries due to abnormalities in the composition, flow and vascular wall of the blood. This term is more related with venous thrombosis (VT): deep venous thrombosis (DVT) and pulmonary embolism (PE). VT is a serious disease with an annual age-dependent incidence of 1-3 individuals per 1000 per year (Naess et al., 2007), with a thirty da case-fatality rate 6.4% after first event and this rate is twice as high in PE than for DVT 4.6%, (Naess et al., 2007). VT is a complex and multifactorial disease both acquired and genetic is involved in the development of the disease. Acquired factors as surgery, immobilization, trauma, oral contraceptive or hormone replacement therapy use, pregnancy, malignancy and advance age (Koenderman and Reitsma, 2011)

A thrombophilia state in an individual is determined by conditions or individual risk factors. However, clinical studies have identified specific factors with statistically significant effects that are common among patients with recurrent thrombotic events. For example, for cardiovascular disease (CVD), well-known independent risk factors include advanced age, male gender and having relatives with a history of the CVD at an early age, smoking, hyperhomocysteinemia, diabetes mellitus, hypertension and / or dyslipidemia (Balleisen L, et al., 1985; De Stephano V,2000, Reiner A. et al., 2001) These risk factors are associated with the different clinical manifestations and some can be modified or attenuated, while others cannot. In recent decades, we have witnessed the description of "new" candidate vascular risk factors, many of which are based on measuring the levels of various substances in biological fluids or on polymorphisms and gene mutations, such as the MTHFR C677T (rs1801133) polymorphism.

The MTHFR C677T (Rs1801133) Polymorphism and Hyperhomocysteinemia

Methylenetetrahydrofolate reductase (MTHFR) is an enzyme encoded by a gene located on chromosome 1p36.3. This gene has a size of 2.2 kilobases (kb) and consists of 11 exons (Goyette et al., 1998). In humans, the product of this gene is a protein of 77 kilodaltons (kDa) that catalyzes the irreversible conversion of 5,10-methylenetetrahydrofolate to 5-methyltetrahydrofolate, the major circulating form of folate (Botto and Yang, 2000). This form of folate participates in the transfer of one carbon atom during the synthesis of nucleotides, the synthesis of S-adenosylmethionine and methylation of DNA, proteins, neurotransmitters and phospholipids (Botto and Yang, 2000). Furthermore, it also acts as a donor of methyl groups on primary methylation of homocysteine to methionine, catalyzed by the enzyme methionine synthase (MS) (Botto and Yang, 2000).

The MTHFR enzyme activity helps maintain reserves of 5-methyltetrahydrofolate and methionine and negatively regulates circulating plasma homocysteine concentration (Botto and Yang, 2000). Homocysteine levels can increase due to environmental factors such as smoking, low folate and vitamin B12 intake and related genetic polymorphisms in genes encoding enzymes or transport proteins (Strandhagen E, et al.,2004).

Excess homocysteine can be harmful to developing tissues (Spotila et al., 2003) and has been associated with CVD (Kang et al., 1991), stroke (Bostom et al. 1999), birth defects (Botto and Yang, 2000) and postmenopausal depression (Slopien et al., 2008) among others.

Defects in the MTHFR enzyme have also been linked to VT (Arruda VR et al., 1977; Cataneo et al., 1997), Alzheimer's disease (Anello G et al., 2004), some types of cancer (Curtin K, et al., 2004), pregnancy complications (Vollset et al., 2000) and neural tube defects (Holt FA et al., 1998). The latter condition has been one of the most widely studied consequences of this deficiency and is one of the most common birth defects worldwide (Botto and Yang, 2000).

Variants for the MTHFR Gene

Different single nucleotide polymorphisms (SNPs) in the sequence of the MTHFR gene alter the affinity of the enzyme for its substrate, 5,10-methylenetetrahydrofolate (Botto and Yang, 2000; Wu et al., 2009). The most frequent polymorphisms are MTHFR SNPs causing the change of one amino acid for another in the protein chain. These are the change of adenine (A) for cytosine (C) at position 1298 of the gene (A1298C), and of cytosine (C) for thymine (T) at position 677 of the gene (C677T). Both SNPs cause a reduction of MTHFR enzyme activity of 50-60% of the normal levels when in individual homozygous form (Kluijtmans LAJ et al., 1996; Vizcaino G et al., 2001; Rallidis LS et al., 2008). Furthermore, it appears that the presence of both SNPs in heterozygous form also reduces enzyme activity in similar percentages. This activity can also be reduced in situations of drastically folate-deficient diet.

Among the SNPs, the variant most often associated with the disorders of folate metabolism is the C677T. This polymorphism, whose consequence is the substitution of an alanine for a valine residue, reduces the activity of the enzyme and increases its thermolability (Froost et al., 1995). The C677T polymorphism can be detected in amniotic fluid and blood (Botto and Yang, 2000) through polymerase chain reaction (PCR) and restriction fragment analysis, since the SNP creates a site for the restriction enzyme HinfI (Frosst et al., 1995; Botto and Yang, 2000).

Interference with the function of the MTHFR enzyme and its co-substrate in the remethylation of homocysteine, methionine, so that the action of the enzyme decreases for any reason (polymorphisms, cofactors or lack of reaction), results in an increase of homocysteine levels (Frosst et al., 1995; Kluijtmans LAJ et al., 1997; Holmes MV et al., 2011). The 677TT homozygote exhibits approximately 30% of the in vitro activity of wild-type MTHFR 677CC, whereas the heterozygous genotype 677CT has about 65% of the enzyme activity of the wild type (Frosst et al., 1995). Thus, homozygosity for the 677T allele is associated with high homocysteine levels, predominantly in individuals with low folate plasma levels (Vizcaino G et al., 2001).

The MTHFR 677T allele is present in 23,7-37% of the Caucasian population in Europe, 30,5-47,5% of the Hispanic population, 8,3-14,6% of the African-American population, and, in a homozygous state, in 11% of the Australian population (Franco RF et al., 1998, Herrmann FH et al., 1999).

This polymorphism is autosomal with incomplete dominance (Frosst et al., 1995; Botto and Yang, 2000). Many factors interact with the function of the variant enzyme. The homozygous 677TT genotype can cause a significantly increased risk of coronary heart disease in the absence of group B vitamins and / or folate, as these are co-factors in the metabolic reaction (Radillis LS et al., 2008; Holmes et al., 2011). It has also been associated with all variants of TE, both arterial and venous, and other diseases such as dementia, certain types of tumors, and migraine (Boston AG, et al., 1999; De Stephano et al., 2000; Anello G et al., 2004; Curtin K et al., 2004). It can be stated that this variant allele is a disease-associated polymorphism in humans.

In populations in which there is a high frequency of folate deficiency, the determination of the MTHFR C677T SNP will identify a population group prone to developing a major and readily preventable cardiovascular risk factor such as hyperhomocysteinaemia.

Hyperhomocysteinemia is the most common clinical feature associated with the presence of this MTHFR polymorphism. Homocysteine is an amino acid resulting from the demethylation of methionine acquired in the diet by protein intake. Since 1976, homocysteine is known to damage the vascular matrix by oxidative mechanisms, reducing endothelial antithrombotic action and promoting the proliferation of vascular smooth muscle, being therefore favorable for atherosclerosis (Morita H et al., 1997; Lloyd M and Taylor Jr, 2003; Rallidis LS et al., 2008).

Hyperhomocysteinemia is an independent risk factor for CVD, coronary thrombosis and death (Lloyd M & Taylor Jr, 2003; Rallidis LS et al., 2008). This factor that has been identified as contributing not only to developing atherosclerosis but also to producing a pro-coagulant state in venous blood (Arruda VR, et al., 1997; Marosi K, et al., 2012)

Among the main causes of hyperhomocysteinemia are genetic factors such as polymorphisms in enzymes involved in its metabolism, most importantly the MTHFR C677T SNP because of its frequency, in combination with vitamin B12, vitamin B6 and folic acid deficiencies, because of their aforementioned role as cofactors in these metabolic pathways (Botto and Yang, 2000; Holmes MV et al., 2011). Indeed, the main factors affecting homocysteine concentrations are low folate intake and the MTHFR C677T SNP (Botto and Yang, 2000; Vizcaino G et al., 2001).

Studies are contradictory as to whether the sole presence of the risk allele without hyperhomocysteinemia is sufficient to increase the risk of thrombosis (Lloyd M & Taylor Jr, 2003; Rallidis LS et al., 2008). However, the situation seems to be clearer in the presence of other risk factors and DM, since the presence of the 677T allele in homozygous or heterozygous form increased

CVD risk without their necessarily being any hyperhomocysteinaemia or folate deficiency.

Given that in Costa Rica there is a high prevalence of the MTHFR 677T allele in homozygous form (29%) (Hermann FH et al., 2001; Salazar-Sanchez L., 2011), and that 35% of these people have risk homocysteine blood levels (i.e., 10 to 15 μmol/L) and 4% have hyperhomocysteinemia (levels greater than 15 μmol / L) (Monge-Rojas et al., 2005). This is important to assess the relationship between this polymorphism and TE in this country.

A protective factor for this condition in Costa Rica is the enrichment of rice, a common food in Costa Rica, with folic acid. This measure, established by an executive decree by the Presidency and the Ministry of Health in 2006 (decree number 30 031-S) (14), is likely to attenuate the effects of the polymorphism, as has been observed in other populations where, after such measures, homocysteine levels in the population, decrease (Tsai et al., 2008).

It is then important to consider this factor, since, according to Kaul (cited by Rallidis, LS et al., 2008), prescribing vitamin supplements can reverse hyperhomocysteinemia and could thus reduce cardiovascular risk. However, the latter has not been proven.

Since 1997, the Costa Rican Social Security Fund (CCSS) is able to analyze the MTHFR C677T SNP for its patients through the Center for Research in Hematology and Related Disorders (CIHATA), but the role of this polymorphism in the context of thrombotic events remains unknown for this country.

By assessing the individual's genotype in combination with other risk factors, the patients may be amenable to treatment and individualized approaches. Thus, the objective of this research was to study the prevalence and to evaluate the effects of known risk factors and of this polymorphism on vascular risk among Costa Rican women with thrombotic events.

Materials and Methods

Subjects

The C677T MTHFR (rs1801133) polymorphism and thrombosis risk factors were studied in 149 female patients with primary episodes of TE, including pulmonary embolism (PE), deep venous thrombosis (DVT), myocardial infarction (MI) or stroke. The patients were admitted to Social Security Hospitals in Costa Rica.

TE was diagnosed by ultrasonography and/or venography. The diagnosis of MI was based on ischemic chest symptoms, typical electrocardiographic (ECG) changes, and elevation of serum creatine kinase and its MB isoenzyme to more than twice the upper reference value limit.

Coronary angiography was performed in the patients. The severity of coronary atherosclerosis was determined by the number of coronary arteries with stenosis of more than 50 percent of the luminal diameter. Patients were included irrespective of concomitant risk factors for thrombosis such diabetes, hypercholesterolemia and smoking.

A complete clinical summary, with emphasis on personal and family history for MI, TE and stroke, and cardiovascular risk factors was obtained from all subjects by a specially trained staff. A subject was considered to have diabetes or hypercholesterolemia when he or she was receiving specific medications to treat these conditions and/ or when there was an established diagnosis of each disease. Information concerning with smoking habits, family history of CVD, use of oral contraceptives and body mass index (BMI) was also obtained for all subjects. Women with BMI >26 kg/m^2 were considered to be obese. Only subjects with history of regular cigarette consumption were included as smokers.

Healthy subjects (hospital and university staff, students and blood donors), without a history of TE and matched to the patients (age and sex) were selected for the control group. All data concerning demographic characteristics and the presence of major risk factors for TE o CVD were collected by the physicians.

Local ethics committees of participating institutions approved this study. All participants gave informed consent according to a protocol approved by the University of Costa Rica Human Subjects Committee and participating hospitals.

DNA Extraction and Polymorphism Determination

Blood samples were collected into tubes containing 1.7mM EDTA-K3. DNA was isolated from peripheral blood according to standard protocols (Miller et al., 1988). For some analyses blood samples soaked onto filter paper cards from the probands were used for polymerase chain reaction (PCR) as described previously (Herrmann et al., 1999).

Amplification was carried out on 50-μL volume samples in a Perkin Elmer-Cetus thermal cycler. Genotyping of C677T MTHFR, were performed by PCR amplification of each of the target alleles from genomic DNA followed by restriction digestion with each of corresponding enzyme HinfI (Frosst et al.,1995; Herrmann et al., 1999).

Data Analysis

Statistical analysis was performed by the Statistical Package for the Social Sciences (SPSS) Version 19. To compare the basic characteristics, odds ratio (ORs) with 95% confidence intervals (CIs) was calculated and test for dichotomized variables. The means of continuous variables was evaluated with ANOVA or Kruskal Wallis test. The observed numbers of the polymorphism genotypes were compared with those expected for a population in Hardy-Weinberg equilibrium using the Chi^2 test. To assess the association between genotypes and MI, VT or stroke, ORs with 95% CIs was calculated. Adjustment was made for the confounding effects of dichotomized and continuous variables. The presence of interactions between traditional and genetic factors was estimated by stratified analysis. Multiple logistic regression analysis was also used in order to examine the relationships between variables. Statistical significance was taken as P<0,05.

Results

Traditional Risk Factors

The demographic characteristics and prevalence of traditional risk factors for thrombosis among patients and control subjects are present in the total group.

The mean ages for cases and controls were 45,0 (± 18,5) years and 54,0 (± 21,8) years, respectively. Of note, 36,6% of the cases were younger than 50 years; these subjects were considered for following analyses as the younger group. Also, 75,4% of the cases were older than 50 years; these subjects were considered as the older age group.

Table 1. Distribution of the MTHFR C677T genotypes among cases and controls

MTHFR 677C>T	Cases n (%)	Controls n (%)	p
677 CC	35 (23,5)	46 (40,7)	0,004
677CT	71 (47,7)	39 (34,5)	0,04
677 TT	43 (28,9)	28 (24,8)	0,55
Total	149 (100)	113 (100)	

p is significant <0,05

Of the traditional risk factors examined, the presence of obesity was significantly different (p=0,006) between the total cases (25,2 ± 4,9) and the control group (23,7 ± 4,1), also followed in decreasing order by use of oral contraceptives (p=0,003), family history of TE (p=0,002) and levels of fibrinogen (p=0,005) in the total group.

In addition, the prevalence of the *MTHFR* polymorphism was a significantly different between the groups (p=0,001) and in Table 1, is present the different value between the genotypes in cases and controls (677T:Wt; 677CT:Hz and 677TT:Ho).

Interaction of Combined Traditional TE Risk Factors in Groups of Cases and Controls by Age

A stratified analysis was performed to explore the interaction of between the age groups (age 50 or over and age under 50) and the risk factors. The results showed that hypercholesterolemia, diabetes mellitus, and elevated levels of fibrinogen were present in the younger group as risks factors. Family history of TE was statistically significantly associated among the older female group.

Median values of total fibrinogen were significantly higher in the cases compared with the control group. The main results of these analyses are given in Table 2.

Table 2. Demographic characteristics and prevalence of risk factors for thrombotic disease stratified by age groups among cases and controls

Variable/ Risk Factor	Cases n=149	Controls n=113	Odds Ratio (95% CI)	p
Age				
<50 years	36,6 ± 8,2	34,7 ± 10,5	N.A	0,3
≥50 years	75,4 ± 11,4	71,4 ± 12,8		0,14
BMI (kg/m^2)				
<50 years	24,5 ± 3,8	22,1 ± 2,7	N.A	0,000
≥50 years	27,6 ± 7,1	25 ± 4,7		0,066
Smoking, %				
<50 years	116	52		
Yes	16 13,8%	0 0%	N.A.	0,005
No	100 86,2%	52 100%		
≥50 years	33	61		
Yes	03 9,1%	10 16,4%	0,51 (0,13 – 2,1)	0,33
No	30 90,9%	51 83,6%		
Fibrinogen (mg/dL)				
<50 years	307,6 ± 114,6	257,8 ± 74,8	N.A	0.002
≥50 years	388,2 ± 167	297 ± 78,5		0,17
Diabetes mellitus, %				
<50 years	19	52		
Yes	09 47,4%	0 0%		0,04
No	10 52,6%	52 100%	N.A	
≥50 years	33	61		0,33
Yes	03 9,1%	10 16,4%	0,51 (0,13 – 2)	
No	30 90,9%	51 83,6%		
Family history				
<50 years	116	52		
Yes	40 34,5%	12 23,1%	1,7 (0,8 – 3,7)	0,14
No	76 65,5%	40 76,9%		
≥50 years	33	61		
Yes	11 33,3%	7 11,5%	3,8 (1,3 – 11,2)	0,01
No	22 66,7%	54 88,5%		

Table 2. (Continued)

Variable/ Risk Factor	Cases n=149	Controls n=113	Odds Ratio (95% CI)	p
Hypercholesterolemia				
<50 years	116	52		
Yes	33 28,4%	04 7,7%	4,8 (1,5 – 14,3)	0,003
No	83 71,6%	48 92,3%		
≥50 years	23	32	N.A.	0,13
Yes	01 4,3%	0 0%		
No	22 95,7%	32 100%		
Oral contraceptives*				
<50 years	114	52		
Yes	19 16,7%	03 5,8%	3,3 (0,9 – 11,6)	0,05
No	95 83,3%	49 94,2%		0,23
≥50 years	8	61		
Yes	1 12,5%	2 3,3%	4,2 (0,3 – 52,6)	
No	7 87,5%	59 96,7%		

Age, BMI and fibrinogen are expressed as mean ± standard deviation. On the remaining rows, the values denote numbers of cases or controls followed by percentage of the total group. Obesity: BMI ≥ 26 kg/m^2. Odds Ratio, 95%CI denotes confidence interval. **p** is significant <0,05.

Prevalence of the C677T MTHFR Genetic Polymorphism

The genotype distribution was in Hardy-Weinberg equilibrium in both groups. The results of the prevalence of the C677T MTHFR polymorphism are given in Table 3. Briefly, a significant difference in the prevalence was found between the overall age group (Table 1). However, in the stratified analysis it was as risk factor in the ≥50 years; old group.

A stratified analysis was performed to explore the interaction between each of the MTHFR C677T genotypes and the traditional risk factors. In the model of the logistic regression and stratified analysis according to age, the importance of the co-occurrences of some of the genotypes and the major risk factors (obesity, p=0,004; hypercholesterolemia p=0,003, use of oral contraceptives, p=0,05; and fibrinogen levels, p=0,002) were detected in the <50 years old group and family history (p=0,01) in the older group >50 years old.

Table 3. Prevalence of the *MTHFR* C677T polymorphism between the case and control groups and stratified by age.

Variable/ Risk Factor	Cases n=149	Controls n=113	Odds Ratio (95% CI)	p
MTHFR	n=116	n=52		
<50 years	Ho 35 30,2% Hz 53 45,7% Wt 28 24,1%	Ho 16 30,8% Hz 19 36,5% Wt 17 32,7%	N.A.	0,43
≥50 years	n=33 Ho 8 24,2% Hz 18 54,5% Wt 7 21,2%	n=61 Ho 12 19,7 Hz 20 32,8 Wt 29 47,5		0,037

The values denote numbers of cases or controls followed by percentage of the total group.

Odds Ratio, 95%CI denotes confidence interval. **p** is significant <0,05.

Conclusion

Thrombotic diseases develop as the result of multiple interactions between non-genetic and genetic risk factors. The known risk factors played an important role as predictors in the development of the thrombotic diseases in the present female case-control study. The most important non-genetic risk factors found among the female patients are: age, hypercholesterolemia, diabetes mellitus, use of oral contraception, obesity, and fibrinogen levels. Moreover, the stratified effect of some of these factors according to the age of the patients is relevant for clinical risk assessment.

In a large multicenter case-control study of thrombosis no association between MTHFR 677T homozigosity and arterial disease was found (pooled OR 1,1, 95%CI 0,9-1,4) (Brattström et al., 1998). The reasons given for the lack of association included nutritional or genetic differences between the populations of this study and those of others (Abbate et al., 1998; Lane and Grant, 2000). This is interesting, in the context of the high frequency of homozygosity of the variant (T) allele in the present Costa Rican female study as compared with Caucasian populations (Herrmann FH et al., 1999; Herrmann FH et al., 2000) and its significantly higher prevalence among the cases versus controls in the overall cohort. Future research in genetics for VT and other multicausal diseases will be based on the new technologies for study the genetic architecture and the specific pathways that are important in the development of the personalized prediction and individual management.

In the present study, an increased risk for thrombosis was found in the older age group with MTHFR 677C>T polymorphism and the major risk factors (hypercholesterolemia p=0,003, use of oral contraceptives, p=0,05; and fibrinogen levels, p=0,002) were detected in the <50 years old group and family history (p=0,01) and obesity (p=0,004) in the older group >50 years old. The small numbers of carriers of these risk factors require a note of caution on any conclusion. Further studies with more patients are necessary for final conclusions for these interactions to be made. However, it is clear that the high prevalence of MTHFR T allele may participate as a risk factor for thrombosis in the older female group.

There has been ongoing discussion on the possibility that MTHFR genotypes could affect the methylation capacity of the estrogen receptor (Slopien et al., 2008). Evidence on the interaction between estrogen status, homocysteine concentration and MTHFR polymorphism and their effect on hormone replacement therapy has been reported (Ottaviano YL et al., 1994). Variations between the concentration of homocysteine among women of different ages and lifestyles that are consistent with effects attributable to estrogen status have been shown (Curtin K, et al., 2004). It seems therefore important to understand if the MTHFR 677TT genotype plays a role as risk factor for thrombosis either in pre or in postmenopausal women (Slopien et al., 2008).

Taken together, the present data suggest that MTHFR C677T genotype may be an important factor in the life of female patients at risk of developing TE or CVD. Folic acid supplementation of foods is necessary (and mandatory in Costa Rica) before and during women's reproductive phase. However, the data presented here suggests that a case for efforts to ensure a good intake of this vitamin in the postmenopausal phase can be made, especially if the high prevalence of the MTHFR 677T homozygosity and of classic risk factors in the Costa Rican population are taken into account. Larger additional studies among women with this genetic and environmental background looking at the combined effect of the MTHFR 677C>T polymorphism and traditional risk factors for thrombosis must be performed for final conclusions to be drawn.

References

Abbate R, Sardi I, Pepe G, Marcucci R, Brunelli T, Prisco D, Fatini C, Capanni M, Simonetti I, Gensini GF. The high prevalence of thermolabile 5-10 methylenetetrahydrofolate reductase (MTHFR) in Italians is not associated to an increased risk for coronary artery disease. *Thromb Haemost* 1998; 79:727-730.

Anello G, Guéant-Rodríguez RM, Bosco P, Guéant JL, Romano A, Namour B, Spada R, Caraci F, Pourié G, Daval JL, Ferri R. Homocysteine and methylenetetrahydrofolate reductase polymorphism in Alzheimer's disease. *Neuroreport*. 2004 Apr 9;15(5):859-861.

Araya M, Guzmán S. Evolución de la Mortalidad por Enfermedad Isquémico del Corazón e Infarto Agudo del Miocardio en Costa Rica, 1970-2001. *Rev. Panam Sal. Public*. 2004:16:295-301.

Arruda VR, von Zuben PM, Chiaparini LC, Annichino Bizzacchi JM, Costa FF. The mutation Ala677>Val in the methylene tetrahydrofolate reductase: a risk factor for arterial and venous thrombosis. *Thromb Haemost* 1997; 77: 818-821.

Brattström L, Wilcken DE, Ohrvik J, Brudin L. Common methylenetetrahydrofolate reductase gene mutation leads to hyperhomocysteinemia but not to vascular disease. *Circulation*. 1998; 98:2520–2526

Botto L & Yang Q. 5,10-Methylenetetrahydrofolate Reductase Gene Variants and Congenital Anomalies: A HuGE Review. Am J Epidemiol 2000; 151:862-77.

Bostom AG, Rosenberg IH, Silbershatz H, Jacques PF, Selhub J, D'Agostino RB, Wilson PW, Wolf PA Nonfasting plasma total homocysteine levels and stroke incidence in elderly persons: the Framingham Study. *Ann Intern Med*. 1999 Sep 7;131(5):352-355

Cataneo M, Tsai MY, Bucciarelli P, Taioli E, Zighetti ML, Bignell M, Mannucci PM. A common mutation in the methylenetetrahydrofolate reductase gene (C677T) increases the risk for deep-venous thrombosis in patients with mutant factor V (factor V:Q506*). Arterioscler Thromb Vasc Biol* 1997; 17: 1662-1666.

Curtin K, Bigler J, Slattery ML, Caan B, Potter JD, Ulrich CM. MTHFR C677T and A1298C polymorphisms: diet, estrogen, and risk of colon cancer. *Cancer Epidemiol Biomarkers Prev*. 2004 Feb;13(2):285-292.

Reglamento para el enriquecimiento del arroz. (Decreto Nª 30031-S) (02/01/02). *Publicado en La Gaceta Nº* 1 del 02 de enero del 2002.

De Stephano V, Casorelli I, Rossi E, Zappacosta B, Leone G. Interaction between hyperhomocysteinemia and inherited thrombophilic factors in venous thromboembolism. *Semin Thromb Haemost* 2000; 26: 305-311.

Franco RF, Araujo AG, Guerreiro JF, Elion J, Zago MA. Analysis of the 677 C→T mutation of the methylenetetrahydrofolate reductase gene in different ethnic groups. *Thromb Haemost* 1998; 79: 119-121.

Frosst P, Blom HJ, Milos R, Goyette P, Sheppard CA, Matthews RG, Boers GJ, den Heijer M, Kluijmans LAJ, van den Heuvel LP, Rozen R. A candidate genetic risk factor for vascular diseases: a common mutation in methylenetetrahydrofolate reductase. *Nat Genet* 1995; 10: 111-113.

Goyette P, Pai A, Milos R, Frosst P, Tran P, Chen Z, Chan M, Rozen R.Gene structure of human and mouse methylenetetrahydrofolate reductase (MTHFR) *Mamm Genome*. 1998 Aug; 9(8):652-656

Herrmann FH, Schröder W, Altman R, Jimenez Bonilla R, Perez-Requejo JL, Singh JR. Zur Prävalenz des G20210A-Prothrombin-Polymorphismus, der C677T-Mutation des MTHFR-Gens und der Faktor V-Leiden Mutation in Nordostdeutschland, Argentinien, Venezuela, Costa Rica und Indien. In: I. Scharrer/W. Schramm (Hrsg.) 28. *Hämophilie-Symposium Hamburg 1997.* Springer-Verlag Berlin Heidelberg 1999: 305-309.

Herrmann FH, Salazar-Sanchez L, Schröder W, Grimm R, Schuster G, Jimenez-Arce G, Chavez M, Singh JR. Prevalence of molecular risk factors FV Leiden, FVHR2, FII 20210G>A and MTHFR 677C>T in different populations and ethnic groups of Germany, Costa Rica and India. *Intl J Hum Genet* 2001; 1: 33-39.

Holmes MV, Newcombe P, Hubacek JA, Sofat R, Ricketts SL, Cooper J, Breteler MM, Bautista LE, Sharma P, Whittaker JC, Smeeth L, Fowkes FG, Algra A, Shmeleva V, Szolnoki Z, Roest M, Linnebank M, Zacho J, Nalls MA, Singleton AB, Ferrucci L, Hardy J, Worrall BB, Rich SS, Matarin M, Norman PE, Flicker L, Almeida OP, van Bockxmeer FM, Shimokata H, Khaw KT, Wareham NJ, Bobak M, Sterne JA, Smith GD, Talmud PJ, van Duijn C, Humphries SE, Price JF, Ebrahim S, Lawlor DA, Hankey GJ, Meschia JF, Sandhu MS, Hingorani AD, Casas JP. Effect Modification by population dietary folate on the association between MTHFR genotype, homocysteine, and stroke risk: a methanalysis of genetic studies and randomised trials. *Lancet* 2011; 378: 584-594.

Hol FA, van der Put NM, Geurds MP, Heil SG, Trijbels FJ, Hamel BC, Mariman EC, Blom HJ. Molecular genetic analysis of the gene encoding the trifunctional enzyme MTHFD (methylenetetrahydrofolate-dehydrogenase, methenyltetrahydrofolate-cyclohydrolase, formyltetrahydrofolate synthetase) in patients with neural tube defects. *Clin Genet.* 1998 Feb;53(2):119-122

Hunter KA, Garlik PJ, Broom I, Andersons SE, McNurlan MA. Effects of smoking and abstention from smoking on fibrinogen synthesis in human. *Clinical Science* 2001; 100: 459-465.

Kain K, Catto A, Kohler HP, Grant PJ. Haemostatic risk factors in healthy white and south asian populations in U.K. *Thromb Haemost* 1999; 82 (suppl.) 185.

Kang SS, Wong PW, Susmano A, Sora J, Norusis M, Ruggie N. Thermolabile methylenetetrahydrofolic acid reductase: an inherited risk factor for coronary artery disease. *Am J Hum Genet* 1991; 48: 536-545.

Kluijtmans LAJ, van den Heuvel LPWJ, Boers GHJ, Frosst P, Stevens EMB, van Oost BA, den Heijer M, Trijbels FJM, Rozen R, Blom HJ. Molecular genetic analysis in mild hyperhomocysteinemia: A common mutation in the methylenetetrahydrofolate reductase gene is a genetic risk factor for cardiovascular disease. *Am J Hum Genet* 1996; 58: 35-41.

Kluijtmans LAJ, Kastelein JJP, Lindemans J, Boers GHJ, Heil SG, Bruschke AVG, Jukema JW, van den Heuvel LPWJ, Trijbels JMF, Boerma GJM, Verheugt FWA, Willems F, Blom HJ. Thermolabile methylenetetrahydrofolate in coronary artery disease. *Circulation* 1997; 96: 2573-2577.

Koenderman J and Reitsma PH. Geographic and Ethnic differences in the prevalence of thrombophilia. In *Thrombophilia* pp: 1-22 .InTech Publishers 2011: Rijeka, Croatia

Lane DA, Grand PJ. Role of hemostatic gene polymorphisms in venous and arterial thrombotic disease. *Blood* 2000; 95: 1517-1532.

Lloyd M, Taylor Jr. Elevated plasma homocysteine as risk factor for peripheral arterial disease-What is the evidence*? Seminars in vascular surgery* 2003; 16:215-222.

Marosi K, Agota A, Végh V, Joó JG, Langmár Z, Kriszbacher I, Nagy ZB. The role of homocysteine and methylenetetrahydrofolate reductase, methionine synthase, methionine synthase reductase polymorphisms in the development of cardiovascular diseases and hypertension. *Orv Hetil.* 2012 Mar 25;153(12):445-453.

Miller M, Dykes DD, Polesky HF. A simple salting out procedure for extracting DNA from human nucleated cells. Nucleic Acids Res 1988; 16: 121.

Monge-Rojas R, Barrantes M, Holst I, Nunez-Rivas H, Alfaro T, Rodriguez S, Cunningham L, Cambronero P, Salazar L, Herrmann FH. Biochemical indicators of nutritional status and dietary intake in Costa Rican Cabecar Indian adolescents. *Food Nutr Bull.* 2005; Mar; 26(1):3-16.

Morita H, Taguchi H, Kurihara H, Kitaoka M, Kaneda H, Kurihara Y, Maemura K, Shindo T, Minamino T, Ohno M,Yamaoki K, Ogasawara K, Aizawa T, Suzuki S, Yazaki Y. Genetic polymorphism of 5,10-methylenetetrahydrofolate reductase (MTHFR) as a risk factor for coronary artery disease. *Circulation* 1997; 95: 2032-2036.

Naess I, A.Christianen, SC, Romundstad P, Cannegieter S, Rsendaal FR, Hammerstrom J. Incidence and mortality of venous thrombosis: a population-based study. *J.Thromb.Haemostast.* 2007; 5(4):629-699

Ottaviano YL, Issa JP, Parl FF, Smith HS, Baylin SB, Davidson NE. Methylation of the estrogen receptor gene CpG island marks loss of estrogen receptor expression in human breast cancer cells. *Cancer Res.* 1994 May 15;54(10):2552-2555

Rallidis LS, Gialeraki A, Komporozos C, Vavoulis P, Pavlakis G, Travlou A, Lekakis I, Kremastinos DT. Role of methylenetetrahydrofolate reductase 677 T polymorphism in the development of premature myocardial infarction. *Atherosclerosis* 2008; 200: 115-120.

Reiner A, Siscovick D, Rosendaal FR. Hemostatic risk factors and arterial thrombotic disease. Thromb Haemost 2001; 85: 584-595.

Salazar-Sanchez L. Geographic and Ethnic differences in the prevalence of thrombophilia. In *Thrombophilia* pp: 39-58.InTech Publishers 2011: Rijeka, Croatia

Słopien R, Jasniewicz K, Meczekalski B, Warenik-Szymankiewicz A, Lianeri M, Jagodziński PP.Maturitas. Polymorphic variants of genes encoding MTHFR, MTR, and MTHFD1 and the risk of depression in postmenopausal women in Poland. *Maturitas.* 2008 Nov 20;61(3):252-255.

Spotila LD, Jacques PF, Berger PB, Ballman KV, Ellison RC, Rozen R. Age dependence of the influence of methylenetetrahydrofolate reductase genotype on plasma homocysteine level. *Am J Epidemiol.* 2003 Nov 1;158(9):871-877.

Strandhagen E, Zetterberg H, Aires N, Palmér M, Rymo L, Blennow K, Landaas S, Thelle DS. The methylenetetrahydrofolate reductase C677T polymorphism is a major determinant of coffee-induced increase of plasma homocysteine: a randomized placebo controlled study. *Int J Mol Med.* 2004 Jun;13(6):811-815.

Tsai M, Loria M, Cao J, Kim Y, Siscovick D, Schreiner J, Hanson QN. Clinical utility of genotyping the 677C >T variant of methylenetetrafolate reductase in humans is decreased in the Post-Folic acid fortification ERA 1, 2. *The Journal of Nutrition* 2008; 139:33-37

Vizcaino G, Diez-Ewald M, Herrmann FH, Schuster G, Perez-Resquejo JL. Relationships between homocysteine, folate and vitamin B12 levels with the methylenetetrahydrofolate reductase polymorphism in Indians from Western Venezuela. *Thromb Haemost* 2001; 85: 186-187.

Vollset SE, Refsum H, Irgens LM, Emblem BM, Tverdal A, Gjessing HK, Monsen AL, Ueland PM. Plasma total homocysteine, pregnancy complications, and adverse pregnancy outcomes: the Hordaland Homocysteine study. *Am J Clin Nutr.* 2000 Apr;71(4):962-968

In: Venous Thrombosis
Editor: Caroline H. Gutmann

ISBN: 978-1-63117-293-9

Chapter 8

Isolated Cortical Vein Thrombosis

Amit Batra*[1], *M.D., D.M., Rahul Rathakrishnan*[1], *M.R.C.P. and Vijay K. Sharma*[1,2,*], *M.D.

[1]Division of Neurology, National University Hospital, Singapore
[2]Yong Loo Lin School of Medicine,
National University of Singapore, Singapore

Abstract

Cerebral Venous thrombosis (CVT) accounts for nearly 1-2% of all strokes. Isolated cortical vein thrombosis (ICVT), a subtype of CVT, without sinus or great venous involvement is rare. It is often difficult to diagnose due to its varied clinical and imaging features. Hence, the available literature largely comprises of single center case series. The common presenting symptoms of ICVT are focal seizures, vaguely defined focal neurological deficits and visual disturbances. Headache and raised intracranial pressure are relatively uncommon. The underlying conditions which may predispose to ICVT are the same as described for typical CVT. However, rare associations of ICVT include lumbar puncture, Hodgkin's disease, nephrotic syndrome, vasculitis, inflammatory bowel disease and amyloid angiopathy. With a high index

[*] Corresponding author: Division of Neurology, National University Hospital, Singapore 119074, Email: drvijay@singnet.com.sg, Tel: +65 67722597, Fax: +65 68723566.

of suspicion, neuroimaging is essential for direct visualization of the thrombus, localized hemorrhage or small venous infarction. Visualization of thrombosed cortical vein (the cord sign) is observed infrequently. Management guidelines are not well established. However, initial anticoagulation with heparin followed by oral anticoagulation for 6-12 months remains the recommended guideline for treatment of ICVT. The prognosis is generally good with radiological resolution in most cases. In this review, we present the clinical spectra, etiopathogenesis, neuroimaging features and management options in ICVT patients.

Keywords: Isolated cortical vein thrombosis; thrombophilia; venous infarction; venous sinus thrombosis

Cerebral venous sinus thrombosis is an uncommon cause of stroke, predominantly affecting the young population. [1] Overall, it accounts for 0.5-1% of all strokes. [2] The term is broadly applied to the clinical syndrome as a result of the thrombosis of the major dural venous sinuses and/or the cortical veins. Involvement of the cortical veins usually occurs secondary to the sinus thrombosis due to the retrograde extension of the thrombus into the veins. [3] Isolated cortical vein thrombosis (ICVT) is a subgroup of cerebral venous thrombosis without involvement of the major dural sinuses. This uncommon condition is now being increasingly reported. The exact incidence is difficult to determine since most of the available literature pertains tocase reports or small case series. The diagnosis of ICVT is difficult due to the non specific and highly varied clinical presentations in association with a wide range of aetiologies and lack of standardized radiological diagnostic criteria. Hence, this entity is often overlooked and remains under diagnosed.

Historical Background

ICVT was first described by Raymond et al. more than a century ago in the year 1880. [4] This work was later referred by Garcin and Pestel in their detailed description of cerebral venous sinus in 1953. Subsequently many case reports and series have been published, describing various etiopathogenic mechanisms and clinical presentations. For example, Cambria reported a case of isolated thrombosis of the Vein of Labbe after Carbon Monoxide poisoning. [5] Another interesting case of the thrombosis of the Vein of Labbe was reported by Yokota et al. that developed a left temporoparietal hemorrhagic infarct and presented with recurrent transient ischemic attacks and pure agraphia of Kanji (the Japanese morphograms). [6]

The diagnosis of ICVT has largely been based on contrast angiography. Rao et al. performed contrast angiography and found that out of their 11 cases with cerebral venous sinus thrombosis, 2 patients suffered from additional ICVT [7] The angiographic features of ICVT were described in detail by Gabrielsen et al. in 1980 [8] and later by Bogousslavsky et al. in 1996, along with the clinical presentation.[9] Although, numerous case reports and series have been published on ICVT describing their angiographic characteristics, varied associations and clinical presentations, the standardized diagnostic criteria are yet to be established.

Pathogenesis

Like thrombosis in any other vein in the body, the three essential components of the classical Virchow's triad (endothelial damage, stasis of blood and hypercoaguliabilty), alone or in combination, are believed to contribute to the pathogenesis of dural venous sinus thrombosis and ICVT.Superior sagittal sinus, transverse sinus, sigmoid sinus and cavernous sinus are the most frequently involved dural sinuses in cerebral venous thrombosis. Thrombosis of the straight sinus and vein of Galen are also reported frequently. It is believed that thrombosis of cortical veins is usually an extension from their connecting dural sinuses. However, ICVT may occur in isolation in some patients. [10] Isolated thrombosis of the vein of Labbe, that drains the lateral temporal lobe into the transverse sinus has been rarely reported. [11]

Thrombosis of a dural sinus, either by thrombus within it or secondary to external compression, leads to its occlusion. Once a major dural sinus is occluded, the thrombus may extend retrogradely to involve the draining cortical veins. In most of the cases, both mechanisms are believed to operate simultaneously. However, only a localised thrombosis may occur, resulting in ICVT. Occlusion due to ICVT often results in oedema in its drainage area and a venous infarction. This is often accompanied by small petechial hemorrhages, secondary to the back pressure and rupture of the thin walled veins. Occasionally, these petechial haemorrhages coalesce to form a large hematoma. The edema that develops after ICVT is vasogenic and/or cytotoxic in origin. Cytotoxic edema results from ischemic damage to the cell membrane, failure of energy dependant membrane pump and cellular swelling.

On the other hand, vasogenic edema occurs due to the disruption of blood brain barrier and leakage of plasma into intercellular spaces. [2] Often, both mechanisms contribute equally to the localized cerebral edema and various neurological manifestations. These presumed mechanisms have been supported by some histopathological studies that demonstrated areas of ischemic infarction, swollen veins, small haemorrhages, dilated collaterals and cellular oedema. [10,12]

The neurological manifestations are mainly determined by the rapidity of venous obstruction, site of obstruction and the affected venous system (ICVT alone or in combination with dural sinus thrombosis). The underlying mechanisms [13] for clinical presentations include -

a. ischemic infarction and subsequent neuronal dysfunction
b. mass effect secondary to large hematomas
c. cortical hyperexcitabilty and resultant seizures
d. cerebral oedema and raised intracranial pressure.

Symptoms of raised intracranial pressure are common with major dural venous sinus occlusions and rarely seen in patients with ICVT. Seizures and focal deficits are more common clinical presentations of ICVT.

Etiology

The etiopathogenic mechanisms for ICVT are heterogeneous and essentially similar to those for dural venous siunus thrombosis. However, in a large proportion of cases the underlying mechanism remains elusive despite extensive diagnostic workup.

Several studies have reported higher prevalence of ICVT among females. Accordingly, about two-thirds of the adult ICVT adult patients are young females. [14] The most vulnerable periods are last trimester of pregnancy and the immediate post-partum period. [15] A major contributor towards ICVT in young females is the use of oral contraceptive agents, especially the third generation pills containing desogestrol. [16,17]

Hereditary thrombophilic conditions such as Factor V Leiden, prothrombin gene mutation, hyperhomocysteinemia, deficiency of Protein C, Protein S and antithrombin-III as well as dysfibrinogenemia are well known associations with ICVT. [18,19,20] However, these hereditary thrombophilic disorders may not be the primary cause of thrombosis and precipitate ICVT in the presence of certain triggers like dehydration, lumbar puncture or some medication etc. Head injury and lumbar puncture are believed to precipitate ICVT in genetically predisposed individuals. Dural tear causing CSF leak and subsequent intracranial hypotension is the presumed mechanism postulated in these cases. [21,22,23]

Some other reported associations of ICVT include Hodgkin's disease [24], systemic lupus erythematosus [25], bacterial meningitis [26], polycythemia [8], nephrotic syndrome [27] and Behcet's disease. [10] Inflammatory bowel disease such as ulcerative colitis and Crohn's disease have also been associated with ICVT. [28,29] Cerebral amyloid angiopathy has also been associated with ICVT in some autopsy proven cases. The deposition of beta-amyloid in small and medium sized arteries as well as superficial veins is thought to be the causative mechanism. The cause- effect relationship may be difficult to establish, especially in view of the presence of cerebral amyloid angiopathy in nearly 8% of normal elderly population. [26] These patients are believed to constitute a 'difficult-to-treat' group, owing to an increased risk of intracranial bleeding due to oral anticoagulants.

Finally, isolated associations of single cases of ICVT have been described with an asymptomatic cerebral arterio-venous malformation (without any anatomical relationship) [30] and in a patient with clinically isolated spinal cord syndrome who underwent lumbar puncture and intravenous methylprednisolone therapy. [31]

Clinical Features

Compared to the arterial tree with a consistent anatomy and predictable neurological deficits, the cortical veins are highly variable in location and size. This characteristic is responsible for the myriad of clinical presentations of ICVT. The non-specific nature and wide spectrum of clinical presentations in ICVT make the diagnosis difficult. Unless, carefully looked for in the neuroimaging studies, the diagnosis may even be missed, especially when a patient presents with mild symptoms. Furthermore, owing to the highly variable territories of venous drainage, the clinical features may vary among patients.

Specific involvement of sensorimotor areas or other parts of functional cortex are more commonly associated with localizable/distinct clinical features like aphasia, hemiplegia or seizures. These are usually acute in onset but may fluctuate over few days. Headache, a very prominent feature of dural venous sinus thrombosis (seen in up to 90% of the patients) is relatively uncommon in patients with ICVT. [32] Some of the patients that present with new-onset isolated headaches may have migrainous characteristics. [12] Thunderclap onset of headache is rare in ICVT. [33] Only a small proportion of patients with ICVT present with headache in association with nausea and vomiting.

Clinical features suggestive of intracranial hypertension such as papilloedema, abducens nerve palsy and altered consciousness are uncommon. Mild impairment of consciousness including confusion, lethargy may be seen in a small proportion of cases with ICVT. Severe disturbances in consciousness may be related to seizures and tends to be transient or fluctuating. However, a persistently poor level of consciousness may occur in patients with thrombosis of the deep venous system or large hemorrhagic infarcts with significantly elevated intracranial pressure. [34]

Focal seizures with or without secondary generalization are usually the presenting symptoms in majority (40-50%) of patients with ICVT. These are usually secondary to the irritative focal lesions over the brain convexity around the central sulcus. [35] Seizures are usually associated with motor-sensory symptoms. Unlike typical dural venous sinus thrombosis, life threatening status epilepticus (partial or generalized) has not been reported in ICVT.

ICVT may rarely mimic a transient ischemic attack, with rapidly improving focal deficits. [36] This may be related to spontaneous recanalization of the thrombosed vein. Patients with ICVT may occasionally present with subarachnoid hemorrhage. A small amount of blood on the cortical sulci may be seen on neuroimaging in these patients presenting with headache, seizures and focal deficits. [37]

Finally, the clinical picture of ICVT may be confounded by the presence of clinical features related to the underlying prothrombotic state, especially when occurring in the setting of meningitis, traumatic head injury and brain abscess.

Diagnosis

A high index of suspicion is required for the diagnosis of ICVT. The wide spectrum of clinical features, diverse associated conditions and lack of established criteria make the diagnosis of ICVT challenging.

Cerebrospinal fluid examination usually reveals non-specific findings that rarely aid in confirming the diagnosis. It may however help in excluding central nervous system infection or inflammatory conditions. Hence, it is recommended only in selected cases based on clinical suspicion. [9] Similarly, electroencephalography is not useful in the diagnosis of ICVT. However, it may occasionally show focal epliletiform activity or lateralized slowing in in some cases. [9]

The neuroimaging features of ICVT include direct visualization of the thrombus, localized hemorrhage, venous infarction and focal edema. The non-contrast computerized tomography (NCCT) of the brain may directly visualize the thrombus within the cortical vein as an hyperdense structure, typically described as 'cord sign'. [38] However, this sign is not commonly seen. Furthermore, it has a low sensitivity owing to the partial volume averaging effect due to the close proximity of the cortical veins to densely calcified skull bones. [39] The indirect signs of ICVT are encountered more commonly, which include sulcal hemorrhage around the vein or effaced sulcii. [9] It is important to note that even for dural venous sinus thrombosis, the sensitivity of NCCT is low (75%) and it remains a poor screening tool. [40]

Magnetic resonance imaging (MRI) is the preferred diagnostic modality for diagnosing ICVT or dural venous sinus thrombosis. When combined with MR venography, it enables direct visualization of the clot in superficial veins, secondary effects of venous obstruction in the form of venous congestion and recruitment of various collateral pathways. [41] The signal appearances vary on T1 and T2 sequences according to its age of the venous thrombus. Owing to the presence of deoxyhemoglobin in the red blood cells within the clot, the thrombus in acute stages may appear hypointense on T2-weighted or Fluid Attenuated Inversion Ration (FLAIR) images and isointense to slightly hyperintense on T1-weighted imaging. Such findings often mimic a normal flow void, contributing at times to a 'missed diagnosis' in some patients with mild ICVT. [42,43] In the subacute stage (end of first – second week) the clot appears hyperintense in both T1-weighted, T2-weighted or FLAIR images, due to conversion to methemoglobin andhence easily visualized as the MR equivalent of 'Cord sign'. On diffusion weighted images (DWI), the clot may appear hyperintense with low absolute diffusion coefficient (ADC). However, this finding carries a low sensitivity (3-39%) since the clot appears bright on DWI only when it is hyperintense on T1-weighted and FLAIR images. DWI, however helps in establishing the diagnosis of an acute cortical infarction. [44]

The addition of T2-weighted gradient-Echo sequence, which is sensitive to the paramagnetic hemoglobin degradation products, improves sensitivity and helps in early diagnosis of CVT. Magnetic Suspectibility effect (MSE) can be detected in the early phase even before the thrombosed vein appears hypereintense on T1-weighted images. However, the MSE can persist even after upto 1 year and hence, may not always indicate an active ICVT, unless the findings are interpreted along with the results of other MRI sequences. [33] For following the anatomical course of the thrombosed vein, the T1-weighted images and coronal sections are often needed. Furthermore, MRI may also help in excluding other conditions that present with localized cerebral hemorrhage such as vascular malformations, intra-tumoral bleed, arterial aneurysms, cerebral vasculitis and traumatic brain injury.

The two-dimensional time-of-flight MR venogram is often useful to demonstrate the thrombosis of the dural venous sinuses and cortical veins. However, compared to the thrombosis of major dural venous sinuses, MRV carries a poor sensitivity (below 50%) due to the variable anatomical location, variable size as well as slower flow. [45,46] Despite some of these limitations, MRI has some additional advantage of detecting parenchymal abnormalities such as focal oedema, venous infarction, petechial or lobar hemorrhage. [47] Neuroimaging findings in a patient with ICVT are presented in Figure 1.

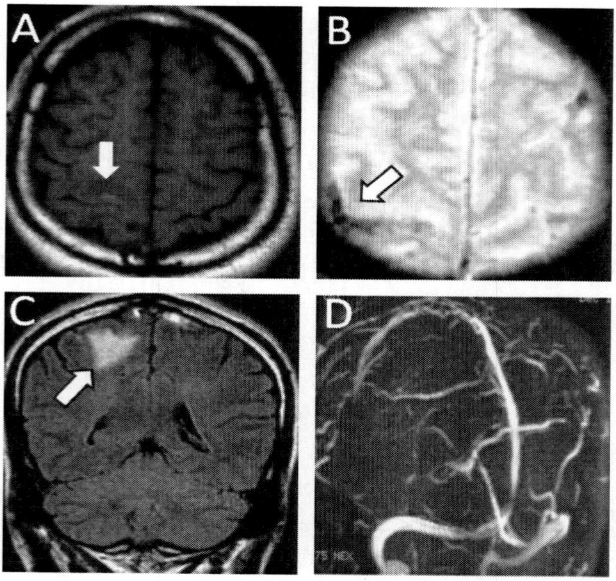

Figure 1. Neuroimaging findings in a patient with isolated cortical vein thrombosis. A hyperintense linear signal (cord sign) on axial T1-weighted MRI represents an acute thrombosis in a right parietal lobe cortical vein (A). Panel B confirms the presence of blood products on the gradient-echo sequence. The resultant venous infarction is seen on the coronal fluid attenuated inversion recovery (FLAIR) sequence (C). Panel D shows normal flow signals in the major dural venous sinuses on MR angiography.

As a result of the above mentioned versatilities, MR imaging has virtually replaced digital subtraction angiography (DSA), previously considered the gold standard, for diagnosing an intracranial venous occlusion. The indirect signs on DSA include delayed or slow local venous drainage, absence of flow signal in the region of a vein, partially filling with abrupt cut off or presence of surrounding dilated cortical channels seen as 'cork screw vessels' or just vascular congestion in the area of the draining vein (so called pseudo-phelibitic pattern). [46, 48] Similar to MRV, DSA is also limited by the extensive variability of size and location of cortical veins in different individuals as well as between the two hemispheres in the same individual. Moreover, DSA relies on indirect signs rather than direct visualization of the vein. [21,49]

Finally, attempts are always made to look for various thrombophilic (especially deficiency of Protein C, S and antithrombin-III, Factor v Leiden mutations, hyperhomocysteinemia and lupus anticoagulant) as well as the vasculitic conditions.

Management

There are no specific guidelines for the management of ICVT and all the treatment recommendations are derived from cerebral venous thrombosis management protocols.

As in other neurological disorders, maintaining a normal body temperature, treatment of infections and good hydration are of utmost importance in ICVT. Some specific treatment considerations in patients with ICVT are described below.

Anti-Epileptic Medications

Seizures may occur in up to 38% of patients of cerebral venous thrombosis. However, there has been no clinical trial that studied the optimal duration and the best anti-epileptic drug. According to the current American Heart Association/American Stroke Association (AHA/ASA) guidelines, it is reasonable to start anti-epileptics early in patients with even a single seizure in view of risk of anoxic damage. The current evidence is strong (class I, level of evidence A) if parenchymal lesions are seen on imaging and reasonable in patients without parenchymal damage on neuroimaging (class IIa, level of evidence B). In patients without seizures, the prophylactic use of anti-epeileptic agents is not recommended (class III, level of evidence C). [50,51] The exact duration for which the anti-epileptic agents should be used is not specified. However, a gradual taper after 6-12 months of seizure-free period is recommended. [51,52]

Steroids

Corticosteroids are used routinely to reduce cerebral edema in patients with mass lesions. However, the use of steroids in reducing vasogenic edema due to ICVT is not recommended. The use of steroids in the ICVT trial was found to be associated with higher risk of death or dependence (OR 1.7; 95% CI 0.9-3.3) at 6 months. [53] Furthermore, steroids are avoided in ICVT due to their procoagulant effects.

Anticoagulation

The role of anticoagulation has been studied in various randomized trials and case studies. Early anticoagulation prevents thrombus propagation and may promote early recanalization in ICVT. The AHA/ASA guidelines, based on all the available data conclude that anticoagulation is safe and effective and recommend early, weight-based and full anticoagulation with either unfractionated (UFH) or low molecular weight heparin (LMWH) (class IIa, level of evidence B). [51] Similar to patients with dural venous sinus thrombosis, parenteral anticoagulation should be followed by oral anticoagulation with vitamin K antagonists to prevent risk of recurrence. In patients with provoked ICVT (those associated with a reversible risk factors like lumbar puncture, oral contraceptive use, dehydration etc), anticoagulation is maintained for a duration of 3-6 months(Class IIb, level of evidence C).However, in patients with unprovoked ICVT, anticoagulation may be continued for a longer duration of 6-12 months, with a target international normalised ratio (INR) of 2.0-3.0 (class IIb; level of evidence C). For patients with recurrent ICVT or first ICVT with severe thrombophilia (homozygous prothrombin G20210A, homozygous factor V Leiden, deficiencies of protein C, S, or antithrombin III, combined thrombophilia defects or antiphospholipid syndrome) life-long anticoagulation should be considered (class IIb; level of evidence C). [52] However, considering the overall good prognosis, long term anticoagulation in ICVT remains debatable. The underlying precipitating factors and presence or absence of microbleeds on MRI may help guide anticoagulation therapy. [54]

Prognosis

Overall, as compared to patients with typical dural venous sinus thrombosis, patients with ICVT have good overall prognosis and complete recovery is observed in nearly 80% of the patients. [11] This may be related to the smaller parenchymal damage, rapid spontaneous recanalization and anatomic peculiarities of cortical venous system. Furthermore, being thin-walled and without any valves, the cortical veins allow rapid reversal of blood flow direction due to an extensive anastmotic pattern. [37] Only a small proportion of patients with ICVT may develop progressive thrombosis and involve the adjacent dural sinuses, resulting in substantial parenchymal damage due to infarction and edema.

Conclusion

Isolated cortical vein thrombosis is an uncommon form of all strokes. Owing to the milder and highly variable clinical presentation, coupled with subtle imaging abnormalities, it is often difficult to diagnose this disease entity. Although, a good prognosis is expected in majority of cases, occasional patient may develop progressive venous thrombosis with considerable parenchymal damage. High index of suspicion is required for a timely diagnosis and appropriate management for ensuring good functional outcomes.

References

[1] Bousser, MG; Ferro, JM. Cerebral venous thrombosis: an update. *Lancet Neurol.*, 2007, 6, 162-170.

[2] Stam, J. Thrombosis of the cerebral veins and sinuses. *N Engl J Med.*, 2005, 352, 1791-1798.

Cohen, JE; Duck, M; Gomori, JM; Itshayek, E; Leker, R. Isolated cortical vein thrombosis: a rare cause of venousstroke with good prognosis after timely diagnosis and treatment. *Neurol Res.*, 2013, 35, 127-130.

[3] Raymond, F. Thrombose des veinesparietales: ramollissement cerebral aigu. Aphasie. Contractures. *Gazette des Hdpitaux.*,1880, 1066.

[4] Cambria, S. Infarctus cerebral hemorragique par thrombose dc la veine de Labbe. *Rev Neurol (Paris).*,1980, 136, 321-326.

[5] Yokota, T; Ishiai, S; Furukawa, H. Pure agraphia of Kanji due to thrombosis of the Labbe vein. *J NeurolNeurosurg Psychiatry.*,1990, 53, 335-338.

[6] Rao, KCVG; Knipp, HC; Wagner, EJ. Computed tomographic findings in cerebral sinus and venous thrombosis. *Radiology.*, 1981, 140, 391-398.

[7] Gabrielsen, T; Seeger, J; Knake, J; Stivill, E. Radiology of cerebral vein occlusion without dural sinus occlusion.*Radiology.*,1981, 140, 403–408.

[8] Jacobs, K; Moulin, T; Bogousslavsky, J; Woimant, F; Dehaene, I; Tatu, L; Besson, G; Assouline, E; Casselman, J. The stroke syndrome of cortical vein thrombosis. *Neurology.*, 1996, 47, 376-382.

[9] Schaller, B; Graf, R. Cerebral venous infarction: the pathophysiological concept. *Cerebrovasc Dis.*,2004, 18, 179-188.

[10] Dorndorf, D; Wessl, K; Kessler, C; et al. Thrombosis of right vein of Labbe: radiological and clinical findings. *Neuroradiology.*, 1993, 35, 202–204.

[11] Bousser, MG; Chiras, J; Bories, J; Castaigne, P. Cerebral venous thrombosis-a review of 38 cases. *Stroke.*, 1985, 16, 199-213.

[12] Sasidharan, PK. Cerebral vein thrombosis misdiagnosed and mismanaged. *Thrombosis*, 2012, 2012, 210676.

[13] Ferro, JM; Canhao, P; Stam, J; Bousser, MG; Barinagarrementeria, F. Prognosis ofcerebral vein and dural sinus thrombosis: results of the International Study on Cerebral Vein and Dural Sinus Thrombosis (ISCVT). *Stroke*, 2004, 35, 664-670.

[14] Cantu, C; Barinagarrementeria, F. Cerebral venous thrombosis associated with pregnancy and puerperium: review of 67 cases. *Stroke*, 1993, 24, 1880-1884.

[15] Martinelli, I; Sacchi, E; Landi, G; Taioli, E; Duca, F; Mannucci, PM. High risk of cerebral-vein thrombosis in carriers of a prothrombin- gene mutation and in users of oral contraceptives. *N Engl J Med.*,1998, 338, 1793-1797.

[16] De Bruijn, SFTM; Stam, J; Koopman, MM; Vanderbrouck, JP. Case control study of risk of cerebral sinus thrombosis in oral contraceptive

users who are cautious of hereditary prothrombotic conditions. *BMJ.*, 1998, 316, 589-592.

[17] Weih, M; Junge-Hulsing, J; Mahraein, S; Ziemer, S; Einhaupl, KM. Hereditary thrombophilias in ischemic stroke and sinus vein thrombosis: diagnostic, therapy and meta analysis. *Nervenarzt.*, 2000, 71, 936-945.

[18] Seligsohn, U; Lubetsky, A. Genetic susceptibility to venous thrombosis. *N Engl J Med.*, 2001, 344, 1222-1230.

[19] Sagduyu, A; Sirin, H; Mulayim, S; Bademkiran, F; Yunten, N; Kitis, O; Calli, C; Dalbasti, T; Kumral, E. Cerebral cortical and deep venous thrombosis without sinus thrombosis: clinical MRI correlates. *ActaNeurol Scand.*, 2006, 114, 254-260.

[20] Mourax, A; Gille, M; Dorban, S; Peters, A. Cortical venous thrombosis after lumbar puncture. *J Neurol.*, 2002, 249, 1313-1315.

[21] Ozlem, KY; Hatice, B; Gulsum, C; Ibrahim, O; Ertugrul, B; Saut, T. Isolated cortical vein thrombosis after epidural anaesthesia: Report of three cases. *Int J Neurosci.*, 2010, 120, 447-450.

[22] Albayram, S; Kara, B; Ipek, H; Ozbayrak, M; Kantarci, F. Isolated cortical venous thrombosis associated with intracranial hypotension syndrome. *Headache.*,2009, 49, 916-919.

[23] Preter, M; Tzourio, C; Ameri, A; Bousser, MG. Long-term prognosis in cerebral venous thrombosis. Follow-up of 77 patients. *Stroke*, 1996, 27, 243–246.

[24] Villringer, A; Mehraein, S; Einhäupl, KM. Pathophysiological aspects of cerebral sinus venous thrombosis (CSVT). *J Neuroradiology*, 1994, 21, 72–80.

[25] Eckman, MH; Rosand, J; Knudsen, KA; Singer, DE; Greenberg, SM. Can patients be anticoagulated after intracerebral hemorrhage? A decision analysis. *Stroke*, 2003, 34, 1710-1716.

[26] Hart, RG. What causes intracerebral hemorrhage during warfarin therapy? *Neurology*, 2000, 55, 907-908.

[27] Schniederman, JH; Sharpe, JA; Sutton, MC. Cerebral and retinal vascular complications of inflammatory bowel disease. *Ann Neurol.*, 1979, 5, 331-337.

[28] Derdeyn, CP; Powers, WJ. Isolated cortical venous thrombosis and ulcerative colitis. *AJNR Am J Neuroradiol*, 1998,19, 488-490.

[29] Rathakrishnan, R; Sharma, VK; Chan, BP. Isolated cortical vein thrombosis in a patient with arteriovenous malformation. *J Clin Neurosci.,* 2009, 16, 856-857.

[30] Al-Hashel, JY; Ahmed, SF; Alexnader, KJ; Ahmed, W. Cerebral Venous Thrombosis in a Patient with Clinically Isolated Spinal Cord Syndrome. *Case Rep Neurol Med.*, 2013, 364869.

[31] De Bruijn, SF; Stam, J; Kappelle, LJ. Thunderclap headache as first symptom of cerebral venous sinus thrombosis. *Lancet.*, 1996, 348, 1623-1625.

[32] Boukobza, M; Crassard, I; Bousser, MG; Chabriat, H. MR imaging features of isolated cortical vein thrombosis: diagnosis and follow-up. *AJNR Am J Neuroradiol.*, 2009, 30, 344-348.

[33] Crawford, SC; Digre, KB; Palmer, CA; Bell, DA; Osborn, AG. Thrombosis of the deep venous drainage of the brain in adults - Analysis of seven cases with review of the literature. *Arch Neurol*, 1995, 52, 1101-1108.

[34] Ferro, JM; Canhão, P; Bousser, MG; Stam, J; Barinagarrementeria, F. ISCVT Investigators. Early seizures in cerebral vein and dural sinus thrombosis: risk factors and role of antiepileptics. *Stroke*, 2008, 39, 1152-1158.

[35] Morris, JG; Fisher, M; Carandang, RA. Cortical Vein Thrombosis as a Mimic for Isolated Cortical Subarachnoid Hemorrhage and Transient Ischemic Attack. *Case Rep Neurol*, 2010, 12, 63-68.

[36] Chang, R; Friedman, DP. Isolated cortical venous thrombosis presenting as subarachnoid hemorrhage: A report of three cases. *AJNR Am J Neuroradiol.*, 2004, 25, 1676-1679.

[37] Ahn, TB; Roh, JK. Cerebral venous thrombosis in adults: the role of imaging evaluation and management. *Arch Neurol.*, 2003, 60, 1314-1316.

[38] Linn, J; Pfefferkorn, T; Ivanicova, K; Müller-Schunk, S; Hartz, S; Wiesmann, M; Dichgans, M; Brückmann, H. Noncontrast CT in deep cerebral venous thrombosis and sinus thrombosis: comparison of its diagnostic value for both entities. *AJNR Am JNeuroradiol.*, 2009, 30, 728-735.

[39] Virapongse, C; Cazenave, C; Quisling, R; Sarwar, M; Hunter, S. The empty delta sign: frequency and significance in 76 cases of dural sinus thrombosis. *Radiology*, 1987, 162, 779-785.

[40] Sharma, VK; Teoh, HL. Isolated cortical vein thrombosis - the cord sign. *J Radiol Case Rep.* 2009, 3, 21-24.

[41] Connor, SE; Jarosz, JM. Magnetic resonance imaging of cerebral venous sinus thrombosis. *Clin Radiol.*, 2002, 57, 449-461.

[42] Hinman, JM; Provenzale, JM. Hypointense thrombus on T2- weighted MR imaging: a potential pitfall in the diagnosis of dural sinus thrombosis. *Eur J Radiol.*, 2002, 41, 147-152.

[43] Lovblad, KO; Bassetti, C; Schneider, J; Guzman, R; El-Koussy, M; Remonda, L; et al. Diffusion-weighted MR in cerebral venous thrombosis. *Cerebrovasc Dis.*, 2001, 11, 169-176.

[44] Idbaih, A; Boukobza, M; Crassard, I; Porcher, R; Bousser, MG; Chabriat, H. MRI of clot in cerebral venous thrombosis. High diagnostic value of susceptibility-weighted images. *Stroke*, 2006, 37, 991-995.

[45] Wetzel, SG; Kirsch, E; Stock, KW; Kolbe, M; Kaim, A; Radue, EW. Cerebral veins: Comparative study of CT venography with intraarterial digital subtraction angiography. *AJNR Am J Neuroradiol.*, 1999, 20, 249-255.

[46] Keiper, MD; Ng, SE; Atlas, SW; Grossman, RI. Subcortical hemorrhage: marker for radiographically occult cerebral vein thrombosis on CT. *J Comput Assist Tomogr.*, 1995,19, 527-531.

[47] Lee, SK; terBrugge, KG. Cerebral venous thrombosis in adults: the role of imaging evaluation and management. *Neuroimaging Clin N Am.*, 2003,13, 139-152.

[48] Duncan, Ian, C; Fourie, Pieter, A.; Imaging of cerebral isolated cortical vein thrombosis. *AJR*, 2005, 184, 1317-1319.

[49] Ferro, JM; Correia, M; Rosas, MJ; Pinto, AN; Neves, G. Cerebral Venous Thrombosis Portuguese Collaborative Study Group (Venoport). Seizures in cerebral vein and dural sinus thrombosis. *Cerebrovasc Dis.*, 2003, 15, 78-83.

[50] Saposnik, G; Barinagarrementeria, F; Brown, RD, Jr; Bushnell, CD; Cucchiara, B; Cushman, M; deVeber, G; Ferro, JM; Tsai, FY. Diagnosis and management of cerebral venous thrombosis: a statement for healthcare professionals from the American Heart Association/American Stroke Association. *Stroke*, 2011, 42, 1158-1192.

[51] Ng, KWP; Loh, PK; Sharma, VK. Role of investigating thrombophilic disorders in young stroke. *Stroke Res Treat.*, 2011, 670138.

[52] Canhao, P; Cortesao, A; Cabral, M; Ferro, JM; Stam, J; Bousser, MG; Barinagarrementeria, F. ISCVT Investigators. Are steroids useful to treat cerebral venous thrombosis? *Stroke*, 2008, 39, 105-110.

[53] Urban, PP; Müller-Forell, W. Clinical and neuroradiological spectrum of isolated cortical vein thrombosis. *J Neurol.*, 2005 Dec, 252, 1476-1481.

Index

A

D

E

F

G

H

I

J

K

L

O

P

T

U

V

W